6

The Critical Issues of Community Mental Health

COMMUNITY MENTAL HEALTH SERIES

Sheldon R. Roen, Ph.D., Editor

Community Psychology Series
General Editor: Daniel Adelson, Ph.D.

Research Contributions from Psychology to Community Mental Health
Edited by Jerry W. Carter, Jr., Ph.D.

Issues in Community Psychology and Preventive Mental Health
By The Task Force on Community Mental Health, Division 27 of the American Psychological Association

Challenge to Community Psychiatry
Edited by Archie R. Foley, M.D.

Coordinate Index Reference Guide to Community Mental Health
By Stuart E. Golann, Ph.D.

Critical Issues in Community Mental Health
Edited by Harry Gottesfeld, Ph.D.

The Mental Health Team in the Schools
By Margaret Morgan Lawrence, M.D.

The Ecology of Mental Disorders in Chicago
By Leo Levy, Ph.D. and Louis Rowitz, Ph.D.

Psychiatric Disorder and the Urban Environment
Edited by Berton H. Kaplan, Ph.D. In Collaboration with: Alexander H. Leighton, M.D., Jane M. Murphy, Ph.D., and Nicholas Freydberg, Ph.D.

The Therapeutic Community: A Sourcebook of Readings
Edited by Jean J. Rossi, Ph.D. and William J. Filstead

Mental Health and the Community: Problems, Programs, and Strategies
Edited by Milton F. Shore, Ph.D. and Fortune V. Mannino, Ph.D.

THE CRITICAL ISSUES OF COMMUNITY MENTAL HEALTH

by
Harry Gottesfeld, Ph.D.

Behavioral Publications New York
1972

Library of Congress Catalog Card Number 76-189950
Standard Book Number 87705-064-3
Copyright © 1972 by Behavioral Publications

BEHAVIORAL PUBLICATIONS, 2852 Broadway—Morningside Heights, New York, New York 10025

Printed in the United States of America

CONTENTS

IV   PREVENTION

V   EXTENDING THE DEFINITION OF MENTAL HEALTH

VI   ROLE DIFFUSION

CONTRIBUTORS

George W. Albee, Ph.D.
Professor, Department of Psychology
University of Vermont
Burlington, Vermont

Bertram S. Brown, M.D.
Director, National Institute of Mental Health
Bethesda, Maryland

Gerald Caplan, M.D.
Professor of Psychiatry
Director, Laboratory of Community Psychiatry
Harvard Medical School
Boston, Massachusetts

Luther Christman, R.N., Ph.D.
Professor and Dean, School of Nursing
Vanderbilt University
Nashville, Tennessee

Shirley Cooper, M.S.
Chief Psychiatric Social Worker
Mount Zion Hospital and Medical Center
Associate Professor
San Francisco State College
San Francisco, California

Elaine Cumming, Ph.D.
Professor and Chairman, Department of Anthropology
    and Sociology
University of Victoria
Victoria, British Columbia, Canada

H. J. Eysenck, Ph.D., D.Sc.
Professor, Department of Psychology
Institute of Psychiatry
University of London
London, England

Harry Gottesfeld, Ph.D.
Director of Mental Health
N.Y.C. Health and
Hospitals Corporation
New York, New York

Henry Grunebaum, M.D.
Associate Clinical Professor of Psychiatry
Director, Family and Child Development Study
Harvard Medical School
Boston, Massachusetts

Lawrence C. Kolb, M.D.
Director, New York State Psychiatric Institute
New York, New York

Lawrence S. Kubie, M.D., D.Sc. (hon.)
Clinical Professor of Psychiatry
University of Maryland School of Medicine
Senior Associate in Research and Training
Sheppard and Enoch Pratt Hospital
Towson, Maryland

Richard Kunnes, M.D.
Division of Social and Community Psychiatry
Albert Einstein College of Medicine
Bronx, New York

Benjamin Simon, M.D.
Assistant Clinical Professor of Psychiatry
Tufts University School of Medicine
Medford, Massachusetts

Thomas S. Szasz, M.D.
Professor of Psychiatry
Upstate Medical Center, State University of New York
Syracuse, New York

INTRODUCTION

The community mental health field is a vague, undefined territory in which all kinds of approaches, services, training, and research with a variety of rationales have staked a claim. For example, a mental health service that treats families together but in all other respects is a conventional outpatient clinic may consider itself to be a community mental health program. Or an educational project that has a parent involvement component or a paraprofessional training program may perceive itself to be in the same domain as community mental health. Even for those officially designated community mental health centers that provide the "essential services" (inpatient, outpatient, emergency, partial hospitalization, and consultation and education), can they be considered fairly equivalent in their community mental health approach or are they more different than similar in their philosophies? How can we judge? What criteria can we use? Until the dimensions of the community mental health field are known and the issues stated, our understanding of the field will continue to be fuzzy and we shall be talking at cross purposes with each other.

This book is based on an empirical study of the under-lying philosophical issues of community mental health. It represents an early but important stage of identifying the dimensions of the field. It is as though one were exploring an unknown area and mapping for the first time the important rivers, mountain ranges, and other topographical features. With a conceptual map of the new, strange land of community mental health one gains perspective on approaches and programs and how they relate to the critical issues of the field. In another sense, bringing together the important issues presents the reader with a descriptive definition of the community mental health movement, what struggles are going on currently, and what may be developing.

This empirical study derived its raw material from the professional literature. Articles and books about community mental health that appeared in the last years of the 1960's were studied, and all ideas, viewpoints, and philosophies were abstracted and a representative group of these were put into questionnaire form. The questionnaire used in the study stands for professional thinking about community mental health at the end of the last decade. The diverse beliefs and approaches to community mental health were presented, through the questionnaire, to 830 mental health workers at eighteen mental health agencies in New York including every community mental health center. Their opinions were subjected to a factor analysis. Six factors evolved.

These factors are the major dimensions or issues of community mental health at the beginning of the 1970's, less than a decade after the community mental health movement was officially launched in the United States. Ideological debates and power struggles are waged around these issues. During the 1970's these issues may wax or wane and new issues may arise. It would seem worthwhile to repeat the study in the mid-1970's and compare the factors then with the factors now to gain perspective as to how the community mental health movement is evolving.

The issues are: Community Context; Radicalism; Traditional Psychotherapy; Prevention; Extending the Definition of Mental Health; and Role Diffusion. The issues appear in the book in relative order of importance as indicated by the research. In the chapters that follow each of the six issues first is described according to the research findings. Then since every issue is controversial and there are powerful arguments both pro and con, an outstanding proponent of both the pro and con viewpoint on each issue was asked to present the arguments in favor of his own point of view. Each contributing author was acquainted with the findings of the study regarding the description of the issue. Some authors were unequivocally in favor or opposed to the issue. Other authors felt their own point of view was not favorable or unfavorable to the entire issue but only to certain aspects of it and restricted their arguments to these aspects.

The final chapter is a detailed report on the research itself. The methods for determining the community mental health issues are explained. The report also indicates how people in mental health in one section of the country, the section with the heaviest concentration of mental health professionals, the New York metropolitan area, stand on these issues and whether their viewpoint is related to their profession, age, sex, ethnic background, type of work, or institutional affiliation. Are the gaps which are often considered to divide people—age, sex, socioeconomic status, etc.—related to community mental health issues?

When the reader has considered the presentation of the issues of community mental health from the empirical and theoretical viewpoints expressed in this book he will have the opportunity to choose if and how he wishes to make his own stand on the critical issues in community mental health. At the very least he should be in a better position to judge approaches, services, and programs.

Part I
Community Context

COMMUNITY CONTEXT

The first issue, "Community Context," is relatively the strongest of the issues and has great importance for community mental health. One aspect of this issue is that in order to maintain a community orientation one should not operate from a hospital or a social agency base. The work should be done right in the community. If institutionalization for an individual seems to be required, partial hospitalization, as in a day hospital, is preferable to full hospitalization.

Secondly, this issue implies that services, in order to be community oriented, must give community people the type of services they say they need, not what the professional mental health worker believes the services should be. The consumer of services determines the kind and nature of mental health services.

Another aspect of the issue of "Community Context" is that the staff operates as an open, democratic community of its own, not as a hierarchical clinical team in which the medical leader is given the responsibility for making decisions. This suggests that in order to work successfully in the community one must first learn to relate openly and democratically within one's own professional unit. The reason for this may be that the kinds of barriers that operate between staff members in terms of power, status, special skills, etc., are similar to the kinds of barriers that operate between staff and community people and overcoming staff barriers will be related to overcoming community barriers.

In carrying out its functions within a community context, the staff tends to use social rather than medical terms, communicating in community language rather than that of a medical institution.

People who are for "Community Context" will be in favor of being, working, perhaps even living in the community, finding out the community needs and responding to them, using everyday terms and having a staff that is a democratic community of its own. People opposed to "Community Context" will be in favor of the institutional setting, professional decision making, and the medical model.

Arguing in favor of "Community Context" is Dr. Luther Christman. Dr. Christman is Professor of Nursing and Dean, Vanderbilt University School of Nursing, Nashville. He holds a B.S. in Nursing, an Ed.M. in Clinical Psychology, and a Ph.D. in Sociology and Anthropology. He currently serves as consultant, chairman, or member of twelve major national organizations or committees and numerous state and local organizations. He has written extensively about role models, organizational structures, and communication patterns in health care generally and in mental health in particular.

Dr. Benjamin Simon, former Chairman of the Committee on Therapeutic Care, Group for the Advancement of Psychiatry, is a practicing psycho-analyst and Assistant Clinical Professor at Tufts University School of Medicine. Dr. Simon believes in a spectrum of treatment modalities in which the psychiatric hospital and/or hospitalization for psychiatric reasons, far from being the anachronism some of its critics believe it to be, occupies an important place.

COMMUNITY CONTEXT

Luther Christman

Health care, particularly that portion dealing with
demonstrable illness, has become so locked into hospital
care that it will take a major shift in attitude and
behavior patterns before other systems will be given an
adequate opportunity to demonstrate their full potential.
Hospitals have become a major support for the fee-for-
service model of health care. Because the economic
incentive is imbedded so strongly in this mode of service,
it will be difficult to start alternative means of delivering
service unless these means serve physicians as well as
does hospital-based care. Having patients clustered
together at one geographic point with all the support
services required to serve a hospitalized or hospital-
related population permits physicians to treat many
more patients in the same period of time. This method
makes it possible for physicians to see many more
patients and consequently to charge a greater number of
fees.

Another powerful group, hospital administrators and
trustees of boards of hospitals, has a major investment
in keeping health care delivery tied to hospitals. The
members of hospital boards usually are persons of
considerable influence in the community and can be
expected to make concerted efforts to keep as much as
possible of the community health services based in the
hospital. A similar type of behavior can be observed in
hospital administrators. Most want to enlarge their base
of operations constantly. As services expand, they are
hopeful that the pool of potential paying customers
increases in size and certainty. Furthermore, such
endeavors strengthen their relationships with the
medical staff, since these activities help to attract more
patients.

Although there may be some economy of scale achieved and the treatment of patients enhanced by collecting all the resources under one roof, there also are some great disadvantages. Hospitals are not internally organized to provide the kind of services patients with emotional problems frequently need. At best, hospitals represent loose holding companies. Seldom are such departments as pathology, radiology, physical therapy, social work, pharmacy, nursing, occupational therapy, and the medical staff working in a harmonious fashion. Generally each separate department is organized to intensify its own inner efficiency instead of seeking ways to make the hospital as a whole an efficient mechanism for patients. When the concept of intense sub-optimization is the *modus operandi,* the staff members from other departments of the hospital may be perceived as unfriendly neighbors and their requests for services as annoying intrusions into the work flow rather than a means of assistance to patients. It is hard to maintain systematic rationality and centrality of purpose in an organization that has the form of coordination without the substance.

As a result of custom, tradition, and vested interest, we have constructed a monolithic agency for health care that may not have the flexibility necessary to adjust to the demands of a tremendously varied population. The stratification of society into so many socioeconomic classes, both within and between the multiple ethnic groups, would not be of such major import in itself if it were not accompanied by numerous other variables. Education, religious beliefs, folkways, superstition, myths, family patterns, recreation styles, communication skills, and political affiliations are types of variables found in an infinite array of singular mixtures. All of these will affect the perception, utilization, and effectiveness of services, particularly mental health services. For example, in some cultural patterns if a person seeks mental health services, it is seen as a disgrace; this is true for instance in the case of the Puerto Rican adult male. An organizational form that is very fluid in its characteristics is required to ride with wide-ranging client demands that are colored by so many subtle overtones. A receptive and pliant form of organization is of utmost importance when the interaction of social variables with mental and emotional stress is at play. This interaction has led many persons operating in the field of mental health to raise serious questions as to whether the medical model for the management of mental health is any longer a viable one.

The medical model appears to be verging toward a more and more untenable and precarious position. The number of persons from the various disciplines, including that of medicine, who are raising questions about the dubious authenticity of the medical model is on a steady increase. The use of traditional medical techniques to put together medical histories and diagnoses and to fashion schema for a diagnostic system has the appearance of being somewhat contrived when attempting to analyze forms of human interactions that are open to so many debatable interpretations. Very little of the scientific technology used in sorting through the possible diagnostic categories can be applied in dealing with the behavior entity that is labeled mental illness. Ullman[1] notes the incongruities and strained justifications observable in the writings of those who wish to cling to the medical model. He then notes that when a person is diagnosed by this method and designated as being of a certain category, the patient is ascribed with all the features of that category. Very broad and vague labels such as "schizophrenic" or "neurotic" replace specific behavior descriptions and the person appears to be treated as an abstraction rather than an individual. Hollingshead and Redlich[2] have documented how this type of labeling of similar behavior patterns takes on a notable bias when the labeling classifications are spread across social class lines.

Furthermore, the kind of treatment formats that come out of the medical model are not always acceptable to clients. The medical terminology that is used to earmark emotional states is confusing and even frightening to many clients. The strange and forbidding terms often seem to stigmatize the client and make him feel as if he were a marked person. The attitudes toward seeking help for emotional problems are as varied as the array of "cultural configurations" in our extremely multivariate society. The perceptual screens that are operating lead to a very selective interpretation about the whole undertaking. The usual diagnostic procedures and accompanying professional activities will be evaluated by patients according to how their perceptions are colored by cultural moorings. The middle class professional person with his finely honed style of professional assessment and planned intervention can be easily misread by persons mired at the poverty level or by the semi-skilled blue collar worker. Great difficulties in accepting or seeking the use of mental health services, especially those that are not community based, can surface when the clients are imbedded in non-English speaking cultures such as the Mexican American migrant workers or our Puerto Rican neighbors.

When mental health services are offered by the staff members of hospitals, the services tend to be underused, to a considerable degree, because of the way these services are bureaucratized. The procedures that are used in hospitals for both inpatient and outpatient care frequently give rise to disenchantment among patients because the bureaucratic red tape is seen by them as derogating or at least exceedingly bothersome and unnecessary. Many of the clients inquiring about care are disappointed by the long, drawn-out procedures, become offended by them, and drop out before any organized treatment plan can be implemented. Much of the underuse of hospital-based services by poor people can be traced to the cumbersome protocols used in giving mental health services. The rigid bureaucratic stipulations make it onerous and at times quite futile to attempt to obtain care except for those who can afford private therapy and thereby circumvent most of the bureaucratic trappings.

The track record that so far has been established by the management of mental health as a purely illness phenomenon has not been outstanding. Even if the behavior that is labeled as mental illness ultimately is proven to be a disease state that requires medical management, the intramural treatment programs may not be the ones of choice.

Models that place the individual in a social context and suggest that the maladaptive behavior emerges from the individual, his role set, and the social pressures that affect him in significant ways, are on the upswing. Scheff[3] offers a social process model that "takes the motive forces out of the individual patient and puts them into the system constituted by the patient, other persons reacting to him, and the official agencies of control and treatment in the society." Szasz[4], by the use of another type of social process model, comes to an essentially similar conceptual conclusion. The behavioral model rests on the assumption that behavior is learned.[5] Persons in disturbed emotional states have learned maladaptive behavior from interaction with their family, with significant persons in their environment, and from faulty coping habits in their interface with the community as a whole. To state the assumption in another way, it might be said that persons in major states of emotional disequilibrium have distorted or very incomplete information about the "real" world. The gaps in information are crucial to normative patterns of behavior and to appropriate role performance.

Therapists having regular appointments in institutionalized settings may not unearth the sources of learned maladaptive behavior with the deftness and certainty of community-based workers who have a first hand opportunity to observe the behavior in the client's natural setting. Since maladaption tends to be situationally defined, it is of critical importance to the client to have help from someone who can become intimately familiar with his entire life space. A more accurate assessment can be made jointly by client and therapist when they both have an anthropological grasp of the situation. Learning or role socialization can be conducted with more understanding by the client after he has been helped to make this assessment and to plot a course of action.

The life space of persons in need of help because of

emotional stress can be examined more searchingly in the social context where the stressors are being applied. The intertwining of social pressures in the environment and the idiosyncratic expression of their impact on the individual client can usually be deciphered more easily when the members of the professional team are sensitized to the issues by daily living encounters in the community. The taking of histories in the supposedly neutral settings of hospitals may not be a neutral experience for many clients. The telling and explaining may lose a great deal of its richness when details are recounted during a medical workup in the outpatient clinics of general hospitals or in those based in state psychiatric hospitals.

Professional persons who are working in the community on a day in and day out basis are more likely to be aware of the fine shades of differences in the dimensions of the problems that are troublesome to the persons residing in the diverse neighborhoods of the community. One is better able to give a rank saliency to these problems, to be opportunistic in managing the problems, to deal directly with dissonance factors in order to reduce disequilibrium, to help overcome sociocultural dislocations, and to reintegrate clients back into their usual life styles when one is in a position to do sophisticated intervention. Patient care or client assistance can be conceptualized in a more unitary form that is process oriented and empirically bound to the community.

Using the community as an arena of action enables the staff members to meet the problems as they are found or expressed and to do so with more precision because the staff has more accurate data. The plan for helping the client can be put together with much more confidence in its elements when all the participants in the planning are equally alert to possible pitfalls. The small staff groups based in the community have the opportunity to be much more cognizant of the total implications of the situation. Thus, they are much less likely to commit errors of omission. Decisions that are not made and actions that are not done for a patient may be more telling and fateful than those that are.

Community-based services are constituted in a fashion

designed to minimize the problems of accessibility and entry into the care system. The heavy overlay of prejudice about the use of mental health services can be dismantled, to a great extent, by the way that the members of the community-based staff react to the overtures of clients. Poor people and the less educated portions of society are tired of professional workers making unilateral decisions about issues that are fateful for them. Most of the team members in the community soon learn to deal with persons who are searching for help according to how these clients express themselves. If the community workers are to survive and have "tenure" in the community they learn that they have to function at the level of the client's perceived and expressed needs and not at superimposed professional definitions of the situation.

The use of paraprofessional workers who are able to supply a linkage between the community staff and potential clients has been a meritorious innovation. Unlike the menial type of work this same class of workers performs in hospitals, the paraprofessionals in the community act as a two-way sensitizing agent. They give credibility to the services that are available by assuring the community residents of the value and integrity of the service. They also act as spokesmen for the clients and assist the staff to remain alive to community issues and to be fully discerning about clients' problems. These paraprofessional workers are especially useful in acting as the contact agent to those persons who have been turned off when they attempted to obtain aid from more formalized organizations.

An advantage of community services that cannot be underestimated is the one of continuity of care. As stated earlier, continuity of care, when supplied by hospital-based services, generally occurs by chance. In the community, on the contrary, it is possible for a worker to monitor the entire care process and remain involved with the client until satisfactory objectives are obtained. This gives the client a sense of security that takes the edge off the anxiety level and lets him use his energies to speed his progress toward health goals.

One of the important components of care is patient

advocacy. The modern complex of highly bureaucratized care arrangements has all but washed out this useful element from the care fabric. Clients seem cared for more by rules, policies, and standard operating procedures than by compassion, interest, and planned use of organizational resources. The members of the staff working in the community have the opportunity to be keenly aware of the dilemmas of their clients and the multivariate nature of the issues affecting each client. It seems to be almost a natural outgrowth of this privy knowledge to assume the role of patient advocate. Many patients do not know how to enter or use the health care system. Unless they have an advocate, they may flounder, falter, and underuse the resources to their own detriment. In addition, the functionaries in most organizations to which the patients present themselves, either in health agencies or otherwise, are accustomed to dealing with that limited portion of the problem that requires their skill or the task activity that is specified in their job description. This comment does not imply that their interactions with clients are not without humane qualities; it does imply, however, that their compassion may be limited to their assigned activities, and as a result, the humane interests may be situationally specific and discontinuous in form. This sort of interest pattern does not serve as the catalytic agent needed to make certain that the client is not overwhelmed by the difficulties of obtaining help in complex, bureaucratic settings.

One of the advantages of being the patient's advocate is that of anticipatory intervention. The professional person taking the advocate role can map out strategies in advance through mental rehearsings of the total situation. This cognitive process may save much reconnoitering time and be valuable in helping to cut into the bureaucratic machinery in order to get at that portion that can be of prime assistance to the client. The more that clients are enabled to have profitable outcomes, the more they are aided to enter and use the system, the more they sense that support is dependable, the more they understand that care is a right rather than a privilege, the more faith and trust they will have in the system. The difficult work of case finding will be made easier when the confidence in the system is established in the minds of potential users. Early intervention for preventive purposes can become a realistic goal when clients seek services when they are in the noncrises stages of their problems.

The dissemination of knowledge about emotional health into the community can be done with more consistency by persons who are seen as rooted in the community. It is much easier to communicate purposefully when a linkage system between knowledge and its use is visible such as is present in the very structure of the professional services of the community staff. Community members can more easily acquire a predisposition to respond to the persons on the community staff because the staff members can use issues in the community to educate the local population and to explain to it the concepts of mental health. In this way the staff is perceived as earthy and knowledgeable rather than as ivory-towered professionals. In addition, the key persons who are caretakers of certain parts of the community, such as school teachers, policemen, employers, nuclear family members, and neighbors can be approached with easier access when the concepts used in teaching are tied to pragmatic issues. This form of teaching-learning is much more meaningful and relevant than the abstract, out-of-context explanations that quite often occur when noncommunity-based professional persons are called in for consultation or workshops.

The members of the community staff have numerous opportunities in the normal course of their work to build a backlog of information into the community network in a cumulative fashion that cannot be achieved easily by professionals based in hospitals. It is superficial education at best, when the attempt to educate the public is done by means of lectures, forums, open houses, and similar transitory efforts. A more useful way is to provide continuous reinforcing contacts that have the capacity to dispel the myths, folklore, and misconceptions about emotional health, using factual knowledge presented in language and in a context that communicates effectively. The community population can become aware of the resources that are available and, more importantly, they can be educated to use them wisely.

Part of the educational process should include teaching clients how to be effectively participating members of the treatment team. The client can be a major contributor to his own progress if he learns how to facilitate the roles of the professional staff and to complement their efforts with his own. In this way, the treatment process can be protrayed as the temporary sharing of a common definition of a situation by persons of such varying backgrounds as the client, his significant others, the staff personnel, and whomever else may be involved. The teaching input must be of a uniformly high quality to accomplish this end and must be conducted in terms the client can comprehend. The client can be an excellent resource for data about the progress that is being made in reducing the stress of emotional states, if he has learned how to identify carefully the fine shadings and nuances in his own internal state and in his interactions with others.

A major, and perhaps the most important, advantage of community-based service accrues out of its advantageous position for developing programs of prevention. There is a whole series of hazards to mental health that exists in the community. Professional persons who are based in hospitals may be vaguely aware of the hazardous conditions plaguing the community. They do not have, however, a knowledge of the inner working of these unsettling conditions and of their direct and indirect effects on the health states of community residents. The workers in the community can become keenly aware of how these hazards interface with the population subjected to them. Thus they have a running start on putting together strategies to cope with emerging and full-blown community problems.

There are two main methods of action that can be employed by community workers to mitigate the effects of these hazardous conditions. The first method, and probably the most widely used, is to try to assist those who are under stress from these societal hazards to develop enough strength to "ride-out" the increased strain and to take the hazards in stride. The second method is more difficult. It calls for eliminating or modifying the hazardous condition by either forming or becoming part of community action programs. For instance, if unemployment increases it may be possible to stimulate local institutions, agencies, and business establishments to assemble a program to try to combat the rising unemployment rate and to find new jobs for the unemployed. If drug use shows a sudden upswing, appropriate community organizations and local citizens can be organized to combat the problem. Community health workers can spot incipient hazardous developments and can get a jump on the problem long before these problem conditions filter into hospital-based staffs. The test of good generalship is the astute deploying of the positive forces and strengths in the community in order to overcome, or at least attenuate, the negative influences. Only by being based in the community can a staff learn to identify what the strengths and positive forces in the community are and how they can be utilized.

Preventative programs will influence direct service programs. Community mental health services generally are understaffed. Efforts invested in tactics of prevention can reduce the possibility of being faced with an overwhelming demand for direct services. Programs aimed at health maintenance (or whatever term is used to indicate a state of emotional equilibrium) are the best insurance against an unmanageable work load.

One of the advantages of community health programs can be observed in staff behavior. The staff acts as its own democratic community. The members of the staff soon begin to realize that the competence of their fellow workers is more important and useful to the work that has to be done than what discipline each represents.

All the mental health disciplines draw from the same basic scientific knowledge that covers the field of human behavior. The free marketplace of knowledge is equally available to all the professions but the role expression of that knowledge may have some differences. These differences spring from the combination of the role socialization process during training and the variations in the depth and range of the kinds of knowledge systems needed to work in each of the mental health disciplines.

Fortunately, the considerable degree of overlap in the knowledge systems of each of the various types of mental practitioners sets the stage for developing shared meanings of the behavior patterns they encounter in clients. It takes time to eliminate the perceptual biases that result from training.[6] Communication processes become much easier as more shared meanings are arrived at as an outgrowth of common endeavors that are mutually satisfying. Small-group interaction facilitates the evolution of shared meaning systems to an extent that is almost impossible in a hospital-based service. This sort of shared understanding for the encoding and decoding of messages with the least amount of "noise" enables the community mental health workers to stay on target and maintain a central focus with much less personal stress than generally can be found in staffs of hospitals.

It might be said that professional roles are inventions of society in order to supply the vital services that can be rendered by specialized knowledge. Society grants certain rights and privileges to these roles but, in turn, it exacts certain obligations. No one professional role exists in a vacuum or grows in isolation. Instead, role behavior grows out of the exigencies of the social milieu in which the role is an integral part in order to meet the expectations of others. The sets of expectations vary according to the organizational setting. When the different disciplines work together in intramural endeavors, there is more likelihood that professional biases will be accentuated because of the constant pressures of others of the same discipline. It is easier to stay moored in one's own discipline, when working in the complexity of a large bureaucracy, than to try to establish identity on a multidisciplinary team.

Despite the plethora of literature on the advantages of

cooperation, the nature of interdisciplinary collaboration frequently appears to be more token than real. Such a situation is less likely to be present in groupings of professionals in the community. The typical sparse staff does not have to pay daily deference to the respective professions of which it is composed. Instead, its loyalty ties are more likely to be of the nature and quality of those seen in primary groups. In the face-to-face relationships that are present, a greater reliance must be placed on others without reference to discipline designation. This state of interdependence can be the nurturing ground for the development of shared power models.

One of the prime ways to serve patients effectively is to share power according to demonstrated competency rather than to allocate it by some power ranking of disciplines. There is as much measurable difference in competency within disciplines as between disciplines. No one discipline, furthermore, has within its training component all the knowledge necessary to deal with the wide array of problems presented by clients. The small groups of professional persons in community-based programs soon grow to appreciate and to quickly acknowledge when one or another of its members has the skill needed to attack a client's problem(s); they can give this acknowledgement without fearing that their own competence has been challenged. In this kind of milieu there is ease of referral and consult relationships. A harmonious rhythm to the work flow can be brought about when each of the members of a clinical team does not have to stand on ceremony and is unencumbered by the restraints of ritual.

One of the desirable outcomes of the dynamics of the group process that can emerge from the interchanges between the community staff members is orderly expansion of the professional role cores of the various participants. There is a built-in professional dominance and hierarchical pecking order in hospital staff.[7] Where there is a marked degree of possessiveness, there also appears to be definite tendencies toward the routinization and splintering of care. The depersonalization of patients and clients is a frequent consequence.

It is far more productive to have the various workers

translate their knowledge into action attuned to the problems of clients than to have workers carefully and methodically spell out the parameters of their respective professions and then strive to stand on their staked-out rights. The use of innovative role expression as an accepted part of the normative pattern helps to generate professional excitement and maximum commitment. Professional persons are more inclined to make substantial contributions when they are not harassed by artificial constraints that impede both the expression of the skills they possess as well as the acquisition of new ones.

If a model singles out one or another of the professions as the base of operations instead of what is needed to serve patients in an effective manner, that model is doomed to ineffectiveness. When the rewards for progress and the attainment of program goals are perceived as joint efforts where the contributions of each member have been truly recognized, it makes it easier to develop a cohesive and professional zeal and morale that is difficult to come by in more monolithic settings.

The mental health disciplines, if its members can be helped to overcome long-ingrained attitudinal sets, have an opportunity to give vigorous leadership to the development of shared power models. These disciplines have a high degree of overlap of knowledge systems and of competencies in general. The situation already exists for considerable extension of the various roles of the present traditional professions. The more the roles are expanded, the more the degree of overlap and mutually shared competencies.

In conceptualizing the best models for serving patients, the chief consideration should be the dimensions of the patients' demand system. The care process is multidimensional, yet it has a basic core. Formulae or ground rules must be established to permit whoever has the needed knowledge and is geographically or psychologically closest to the patient to be free to intervene and assist the patient without being apprehensive about reprisals from the members of other disciplines. This type of model is very relevant to key issues of the day—those of easy acess of the client to the care process and the attainment of professional destiny by each of the staff participants. Thus it holds promise of a greater degree of both patient and worker satisfaction.

The strategy for spelling out the basis for participation by partnership can be agreed upon more readily than endlessly trying to negotiate about the tasks that are permitted or not permitted to be done. The community programs offer a far more fluid set of conditions in which to experiment with this type of model for the reasons previously outlined. The main characteristics of this way of modeling care have been stated in this fashion:

> There probably is no model that is a paragon. .... This being the case, there will have to be variations on the theme of interdependence. Each workable model will have fine differences, but some general principles will be part of all. Shared interpretations of goals and means; a system where mutual expectations can be fulfilled through a process of complementation; facilitation of each other's roles; self-direction without anarchy; and a sense of professional destiny and self-fulfillment are attributes that seem crucial to the successful mobilization of interdisciplinary resources.[8]

Even though the main thesis being promulgated in this essay is the suggestion that the treatment of persons with problems of emotional health can be done most advantageously in the community in which the persons with problems live, there are two noteworthy pitfalls that can have adverse consequences for clients. The first is the developing of too much congruency of beliefs and behaviors between the staff members themselves. Unlike the state of affairs within hospitals that tends to pull multidisciplinary staff units apart, the kinsman-type relationships of the community-based staff may produce so tight a bond that the members are unable to see error in each other. Too much agreement about means and ends hampers a group's productivity and creates as undesirable a social condition as too little agreement. One insightful study has demonstrated this principle with considerable clarity.[9] If one observes a multidisciplinary team that is too congruent obsessing over the discussion of a patient, nodding heads in agreement, and consoling each other in their therapeutic helplessness, it is not too difficult to come to the conclusion that all is not well. A little dissonance injected into this group might result in some therapeutic effectiveness. A certain amount of disagreement acts as a check for error. In order to maintain their sharp cutting edge, the community staffs should have outside review from time to time, have some modest and regular exchange of staff members, call upon outside consultants, and have funds available to visit other operational groups and to attend outside workshops. Interpersonal stagnation can be avoided with suitable precautions.

The other danger and perhaps the most disruptive of the two, insofar as client welfare is concerned, is the taking on of a territorial possessive attitude. There are more persons needing support and care than there are agencies and trained persons to do the job. If all the agencies and workers could be combined in some massive and closely articulated design, there still would be massive gaps in care. It is intolerable to have any group pace off territory and put a professional curtain around it. The community workers need to be as helpful as possible in enabling other groups and agencies to serve the community residents. The members of the community staffs cannot complain about roadblocks being placed in the way of getting services for their patients and at the same time obstruct the attempts of agencies to follow through on the treatment plans that the agencies have for patients. It will take strenuous endeavors to keep all channels open. Professional baronies survive and throw up unassailable fortresses wherever constant warfare is the theme.

Collaboration is attainable with the minimal amount of negotiation when the entire array of care resources is conceptualized as an open system and the resources are made equally available to everyone. While this paragon is almost unattainable, it should be the model that guides the way that organizations, large and small, mold their direction if the best interest of clients is the central motif.

Developing a social milieu to try to bring about an

environment that will enable patients to develop a social "fit" calls for a sophisticated approach. Patients can maintain themselves as productive citizens if the supporting structure is anchored into their day-to-day world. A design of care that (1) can be keenly sensitive to the stressors at play; (2) can generate subtle and unobtrusive intervention at the right time; (3) is capable of fluid adjustment to clients' demands; (4) provides easy access to care; (5) is not locked tightly into traditional models of care; (6) has the capacity to make rapid adaptation to new knowledge; (7) promotes staff collaboration; and (8) can engender user confidence is a major contribution to the management of that wide variety of emotional problems of persons that is broadly lumped under the rubric of mental health. The concept of community based mental health services encompasses all of the above requirements. It has the potential for being of inestimable value in delivering services to troubled people. It is the top choice of the alternatives to care.

REFERENCES

1. Ullman, L.P., Behavior Therapy as Social Movement (p. 498) in Franks, C.M. (ed.) *Behavior Therapy: Appraisal and Status,* New York, McGraw-Hill, 1969.

2. Hollingshead, A.R., and Redlich, F.C., *Social Class and Mental Illness: A Community Study,* New York, Wiley, 1958.

3. Scheff, T.J., *Being Mentally Ill: A Sociological Theory,* Chicago, Aldene, 1966.

4. Szasz, T.S., *The Myth of Mental Illness,* New York, Hueber-Harper, 1961.

5. Ullman, *op.cit.,* p. 498.

6. Chance, E., and Arnold, J., The Effect of Professional Training, Experience and Preference for a Theoretical System Upon Clinical Case Description. *Human Relations* 13: 195-213, 1960.

7. Caudhill, W., *The Psychiatric Hospital as a Small Society,* Boston, Harvard University Press, 1958.

8. Christman, L., Community Resources—The Role of Other Professionals, *Medical College of Virginia Quarterly* 5: 143-146, 1969.

9. Adams, S., Status Congruency as a Variable in Small Group Performance, *Social Forces* 32: 16-22, 1953.

THE VALUE OF
THE PSYCHIATRIC HOSPITAL

Benjamin Simon

There has been a negative attitude toward the psychiatric hospital which even preceded the community mental health movement. It has almost been part of the folklore of American medicine that a psychiatric hospital should be avoided at all times. It has become a slogan to help patients out of psychiatric hospitals and use the psychiatric ward of a general hospital if you can. The current enthusiasm for the community mental health movement has further denigrated the psychiatric hospital and encouraged the notion that the only good psychiatry is treatment in the community. In fact, so strong has this attitude been that the original Medicare/Medicaid King-Anderson bill excluded care of the mentally ill in any institution which was primarily for the care of the mentally ill, but included psychiatric care in a general hospital!

Every innovation in treatment has been followed by bandwagon movements which saw these new modalities (such as insulin therapy, electroconvulsive therapy, tranquilizers, etc.) as the be-all and end-all solution to very complex problems in mental illness. To claim that a community mental health center is the solution to all psychiatric needs is to deprive some patients of needed resources.

I want to address myself to what the psychiatric hospital can and should be and what it can offer patients. I am not referring here to the quality of mental hospital care, wherever it may be, for individual deficiencies should be dealt with as such.

I also speak from the medical model that the mentally ill person is suffering from a medical disorder. I do not

23

deny the multiplicity of factors impinging on this, as they also impinge on organic medical disease. I refer here to problems of society and environment, but I feel that the medical model significantly includes these and deals with them as effectively as possible through auxiliary services such as social service.

There are two dangerous fallacies in regard to hospital care for the mentally ill which are fostered by the community mental health center enthusiasts. The first is that a patient should be treated at home or very near home. The removal of a patient from his immediate community is seen as being detrimental to his treatment. However, the concept of an asylum is not without merit. It offers the patient a chance to remarshal his forces and regain the strength to begin anew away from the very noxious psychic and social forces which have contributed to his illness in the first place. Lawrence Kubie writes very eloquently on this point in his paper "Pitfalls of Community Psychiatry" when he says ". . . Would it be wise to launch the treatment of a malarial patient on the very malarial swamp where he had contracted his illness? . . . Practical circumstances may compel us to launch and conduct psychiatric treatment with the patient residing in his own home and community, but only rarely is this advisable."[1]

The second fallacy which has been fostered by the claims of the community mental health movement is the concept of hospitalization by default; in other words, when all else fails, hospitalization is the final resort. This notion in itself creates strong feelings of demoralization on the part of the patient and his family. It also gives a negative connotation to the use of the psychiatric admission; whereas the psychiatric hospital should be seen as part of the general arsenal for the effective treatment of the mentally ill. If it were viewed in this way it would be seen not as a debilitating social anachronism but as a therapeutic complex for those under stress who have a need for psychological retreat.

The positive reasons for admission to a hospital for psychiatric care are the same as those for admission for general medical care.[2] It is to be recommended when:

1) skilled clinical observation is needed for diagnostic clarification;
2) special medical, nursing, and rehabilitation treatment is required.

The hospital provides an ideal environment in which extended observation can be made of the patient's behavior and his mode of relating to others. Nurses, attendants, and other hospital personnel keep careful notes of his behavior during the day and night, the degree of distress he manifests, his observable symptoms, how he relates to fellow patients and to hospital authorities, and the degree to which he participates in hospital activities. If the patient's distress and symptom picture continue, this suggests deeprooted, intrapsychic conflict. On the other hand, if they abate this is more suggestive of situational problems.

In addition to observation, the hospital setting permits various specialists to be easily brought together. Each can make a unique contribution to the understanding of the patient's behavior. The psychiatrist, through his psychiatric examination, the psychologist, through psychological tests, and the psychiatric social worker, by obtaining family history, together contribute to a more complete understanding of the patient. Also available, when needed, in a hospital setting are neurologists, other medical specialists, and laboratory facilities to help determine possible organic components of the patient's disturbance. These specialized services are available almost exclusively in hospitals and help to determine whether the patient is suffering from a functional and/or organic disorder, the degree of impairment, and the etiology. With such knowledge an accurate diagnosis can be determined and an adequate treatment plan can be formulated.

The hospital offers a multitude of treatment resources that can be individualized according to the needs of each patient. Individual psychotherapy, group psycho-therapy, electroconvulsive therapy, psychopharma-cologic drugs, and occupational and recreational therapy are typical therapeutic procedures available in a hospital setting. In some hospitals therapeutic modes such as family therapy and patient government have been instituted. Milieu therapy has been developed as a formal therapeutic procedure in some psychiatric hospitals but in every good psychiatric facility milieu therapy is in operation whether formalized or not. A pleasant hospital atmosphere, individual attention and continuity of care all provide a therapeutic milieu and contribute to the patient's recovery.

The management of special treatments, somatic procedures, and psychopharmacologic drugs often requires continuous observation. This type of management is best carried out in a hospital with its continuous nursing care and controlled setting. The hospital is also an excellent facility when medications and drugs on which the patient has become dependent must be withdrawn. In still other instances the need for hospitalization is not as apparent. Although a patient may not be manifesting an extreme pathological state, his mental illness may cause severe family disequilibrium. If the resources of the family are extremely strained, hospitalization may be indicated to enable the family to recover its own equilibrium.

There are certain emergency situations where psychiatric hospitalization is undoubtedly the treatment of choice. For example, the actively suicidal patient certainly should be in a hospital. It is the best treatment when an individual becomes a threat to others because of paranoid projections or delusions which result in a breakdown of control. In cases of panic resulting either from acute anxiety or from toxic or psychological reasons, hospital care provides the immediate withdrawal from the environment which this state requires.

Some have criticized hospitals for their routinized, seemingly dehumanized, procedures. Of course, it is true that in any large organization standard operating procedures will be necessary. But beyond this, in medicine a routine procedure tends to be based on good clinical and/or administrative practice and is helpful to the patient. For example, on a psychiatric ward the routine serving of meals at set hours is wise from a clinical and administrative viewpoint. It allows for better supervision of patients' food intake, creates a stable, orderly procedure for patients who may have mainly experienced chaos and disorder in their lives, helps to assure patients that their needs are being met, provides a pleasant period of oral gratification and socialization, and results in more efficient use of staff and patients' time. In fact, the utilization of these good routinized procedures helps create the positive therapeutic milieu of the hospital ward. Many patients look back on their hospital stay as a pleasant experience despite the misery and stress that brought them there.

I would like to address myself to two fields that are related to clinical practice and upon which, to a large extent, good clinical practice depends, and to point out the actual and potential contributions of the hospital. These two fields are training and research. Training is a routine and integral part of most modern hospitals. Psychiatrists and psychiatric nurses as well as many clincal psychologists and psychiatric social workers received their training in a psychiatric hospital or the psychiatric division of a general hospital. In these hospitals the mental health professionals learn through diagnostic and treatment experiences with a large variety of psychiatric patients having varying degrees of disturbance and different types of emotional dynamics. In these hospitals the clinicians receive training and close supervision of their work by senior staff people. In hospital settings young professionals learn about clinical teamwork and the contributions that can be made by other disciplines. It is here that the first lessons about high standards of clinical practice and ethical considerations may first be taught. While the student is receiving his theoretical training in the university it is in the hospital that the budding clinician is learning the application of his art and profession.

The bringing together, under one roof, of facilities, experts of different disciplines, and a variety of patients (no small administrative feat) results in maximum training opportunities for clinical students. Universities are quick to see the advantages of hospital placement and to arrange affiliations between the hospital and the university. The hospital setting, where service and training go on side by side, seems to benefit both service and training. No training lesson has greater impact on the student than seeing a psychiatric principle demonstrated by a patient's behavior. The relative value of a treatment modality becomes clear to the student when he has the opportunity to observe its effects on various patients. On the other hand, for the working clinicians of a hospital the knowledge that theirs is a training hospital and that hospital services not only benefit the patients but also train students seems to further enhance the value of their work and contributes to high staff morale. In such a hospital one immediately senses this spirit in the bustling, highly motivated staff and the intense interest at staff meetings, case conferences, and ward rounds. The availability of patients, facilities, and clinical expertise for training purposes may exist in no other institution to the degree to which it does in hospitals.

Clinical research contributes to the pool of knowledge upon which services are based. Good research depends upon the fulfillment of a number of demanding conditions. Research requires staff that have appropriate technical research skills and familiarity with the type of phenomena they wish to study, animals or humans that are available for study or experimentation, and properly controlled conditions and research equipment for recording or analyzing data. Today most hospitals could fulfill these conditions. They often have staff trained in research methodology, always have clinical staff, frequently are able to enlist the cooperation of patients as research subjects, have fairly controlled conditions (some hospitals even have specially designed rooms where environmental variables are very well controlled), and many hospitals have such technical facilities as electronic data processing. Indeed, a considerable proportion of all psychiatric research is being conducted today in hospitals. Many important studies and their findings have already been reported on such vital matters as the effects of various treatment modalities, staff and patient interactions, patient information systems, and patterns of patient care. These research studies are beginning to influence the policies and practices of both institutions and individual clinicians.

I think that more could be done by hospitals in terms of their research efforts. Evaluation of psychiatric programs is still more the exception than the rule. Patients' records are a rich but largely untapped source of research information. I believe that hospitals are ideal settings for psychiatric research and this should be fully exploited. Hospitals are coming around to this point of view. Initially hospitals were fully involved in providing services, then services and training, and now they are developing research programs as well. This direction holds much promise for the mental health field.

Those who advocate the dissolution of hospital psychiatry in favor of community psychiatry will not cause the tearing down of the psychiatric hospital. What could happen is that much of the progress made in hospital psychiatry will be halted. This could mean that our mental hospitals would again become what they once were, repositories for those who have not responded to other therapies. Since there will inevitably be patients who *faute de mieux* will perforce require hospitalization, the era of custodial care for the isolated and abandoned mental patient may well be reinstituted.

I do not believe that a hospital in itself can have an adverse effect on a patient. Any such effect represents a failure in hospital performance, not a failure in principle. For that matter, the question of performance can equally be applied to community mental health centers. There are too few centers which perform in a comprehensive manner, offering all treatment modalities in their resources—which include wellplanned hospital care. There are too many which do not and ultimately will not because of poor coordination of function and the internecine power struggles which have marred many programs in the past and unhappily will continue to do so in the future. Interestingly, these centers frequently slough off their responsibilities by unjustified commitment to psychiatric hospitals.

What is needed above all is a continuity of medical care in which the psychiatric hospital is part of the total spectrum of resources within a community mental health center in which patients may move freely from one facility to another. I do not believe that the mental hospital should be a substitute for the community mental health center or that the mental health center should substitute for the hospital. Each has its own merits and in each case the combined use of both in an intelligent and professional way is the only rational goal.

REFERENCES

1. Kubie, Lawrence, "Pitfalls of Community Psychiatry", *Archives of General Psychiatry,* March 1968, Vol. 18, p. 262.
2. Group for the Advancement of Psychiatry, Committee on Therapeutic Care, *Crisis in Psychiatric Hospitalization,* March 1969, Vol. 7, No. 72.

Part II
Radicalism

RADICALISM

The issue of "Radicalism" relates to a dissatisfaction with the progress that has been made in community mental health and a belief that rapid, drastic changes are needed. Political and economic implications are considered to be the important aspects of community mental health, as they are for any institution or movement. Those who support the radical position believe that the centers must become involved politically and use methods that reach large masses of people. They hope that the mental health centers will become controlled by community people; they feel that those who currently are in charge are the same professional administrators who have always had a stake in the status quo and are unlikely to make any meaningful changes in community mental health. These professional administrators have not been accountable to the people.

Those opposed to "Radicalism" have a "go slow" attitude. They feel that the knowledge and skills learned in applying mental health in the community have been hard-earned and worthwhile but that the community mental health movement should move ahead carefully, making certain of its ground. They believe that there have been too many undertakings in community mental health based on enthusiasm alone rather than on careful planning and knowledge. They are fearful of some tendencies they see in community mental health that seem to go contrary to good clinical care or the proper training of mental health staff. They feel that the community mental health movement should be concerned with health and not politics. They have serious doubts about placing community people in decision-making roles in the community mental health

33

centers; community people are likely to be unsophisticated and subject to political manipulation.
Opposite sides of this issue are taken by Dr. Richard Kunnes and Dr. Lawrence C. Kolb. Dr. Kunnes has been affiliated with the Division of Community and Social Psychiatry, Albert Einstein College of Medicine, and with the Health Policy Advisory Center (Health PAC), an organization critical of health care in the United States. Dr. Kunnes is a radical in theory and practice. He has written a number of articles on the politics of psychiatry, the radical therapist, and community control of health services, and has participated in confrontations with the medical establishment.

Dr. Kolb is Past President, American Psychiatric Association, and Director of the New York State Psychiatric Institute. He has a lifetime of service in the planning and administration of mental health services and has been active at the federal, state, and local levels in developing service delivery systems. Dr. Kolb sees radicalism as a danger to the community mental health movement.

RADICALISM AND COMMUNITY MENTAL HEALTH

Richard Kunnes

The word "radical" comes from the Latin, *radix,* meaning "root." The radical psychiatrist, psychologist, or therapist, therefore, gets to the root or cause of the issues before him (her) and does something about them.[9] A recent cover of the journal, *The Radical Therapist,* said: "Therapy is a political change . . . not peanut butter." [17] This implies that the root issues the radical therapist deals with are political.

What does politics have to do with psychiatry and mental health? One of the purposes of this paper will be to show the relationship between the American political system and community psychiatry. There are two perspectives by which this relationship can be examined:

1) First, there is the theme that the psychiatric profession and its services are a part of and give support to the U. S. politico-economic system.

2) Second, there is the theme that the U. S. politico-economic system itself is *the* major cause of psychiatric disability. These two themes or perspectives, if accepted as fact, have tremendous implications for psychiatry in general and community psychiatry in particular. I will expand on these themes below.

1. Psychiatry as Part of the U. S. Politico-economic system

The general politico-economic system of the U. S. is capitalism. Just as the economy has historically evolved along capitalistic lines, so has psychiatry. For example, psychiatric services have evolved from the entrepreneurial laissez-faire of the private practitioner to the corporate liberalism of the community mental health center.[11] The new psychiatry in the community is different from the old psychiatry, in that in the case of the old psychiatry the "adjuster" was the psychiatrist alone in his private office. In the case of the new psychiatry the "adjuster" is a team of corporately functioning elites, e.g., urbanologists, economists, architects, penologists, as well as the community psychiatrist. The prominent theories of psychiatry and mental health have evolved from psychoanalysis to modern systems analysis.

Just as our economy and politics have become dominated by the mechanisms of the military-industrial complex, the mental health market is dominated by similar mechanisms. First, there is the emphasis on pacification and counterinsurgency. Second, there is the fact that just as the defense industry is really a war industry, the mental health market is really a mental illness market. Third, both this industry and that market are basically profitless, if run on a large scale, without three major components[15]: war, illness, and money. The defense industry needs war, or a threat of war, while the mental health market needs mental illness—and both need an influx of federal money to stabilize the financial bases of their respective markets. Much of the current intraprofessional feuding is between the old-line, laissez-faire, isolationistic, conservative, and financially independent entrepreneurial solo-practitioner versus the modern, corporately liberal community mental health specialists, dependent on an influx of federal money. While the style of the debate focussed on professional technology and skills, e.g., couches versus community centers, psychoanalysts versus systems analysts, etc., the real issue, namely that mental health programs and priorities evolve not along therapeutically efficacious lines, but along general economic lines, remained undiscussed. Economic principles are more important than psychiatric principles.[6]

No matter what stage of psycho-economic evolvement we are in, psychiatry serves the system and its norms.

Community mental health aims at the systematic subordination of individual behavior to false social norms. For example, look at some of the roles community psychiatry plays in the following settings:

1. Schools. Here the psychiatrist or the community mental health specialist labels individual students or groups of students as "sick" or "problems," and not the school administration or structure or the politico-economic system in which it functions. The psychiatrist's role is to serve the school[20] and not the students. That the schoool is a mindless and alienating, racist and sexist tracking system for the military-industrial complex is never seriously examined. Such an examination calls for a political response, not a psychiatric one. Not to examine these issues is to "rationalize," in the Rand Corporation sense of the word, the school system.

2. Police. Increasingly, police departments are allying themselves with academic departments of psychiatry[5] for assistance in dealing with individual offenders, crowd control, and "conflict resolution." In effect, community mental health programs and psychiatrists, under the guise of "medical methods," serve as public relations experts for one of our most repressive institutions.

If not directly working for city police, psychiatrists and other community mental health specialists will be using their skills for purposes of social control. Thus, a past president of the American Medical Association, along with a chairman of a psychiatry department, jointly call for psychiatrists to systematically collect basic behaviorial data on all U. S. citizens to allow the community psychiatrist to forecast and control "behaviors of populations under a variety of circumstances. Better control of human behavior must be achieved,"[3] they said.

3. The Family and Women. A woman's failure to accept her prescribed roles as a housekeeper, nursemaid, and husband pamperer is explained to her as resulting from her psychological inadequacies as a mother and wife, rather than from the flaws in the instutition of marriage and the family.

Women who are not passive and sweet, but instead are assertive and independent, are labeled guilty of "penis-envy."

Rebellion in the black community is explained away and dealt with as a problem in the " . . . instability of the Negro family,"[21] rather than as a problem in institutional racism and poverty.

4. Industry. Here community psychiatrists are used to maximize worker productivity, as opposed to worker well-being. For example, industrial consultant Dr. Eli Ginzberg[4] suggests to executives that they provide mental health services only for neurotics and not for psychotics, to avoid ". . . throwing good money after bad."

The Wall Street Journal reports that encounter groups for executives were abandoned because the executive became less dogmatic and less authoritarian, and thus was ". . . not the boss he had been."

If not working to maximize worker productivity, psychiatrists can work to maximize corporation profits. For example, numerous psychiatrists "are out in the community" consulting with various Madison Avenue advertising agencies that are in the forefront of designing sexist material to push consumer consumption of worthless, if not dangerous, products.

Elsewhere, psychiatrists are helping corporations diversify. For example, Lockheed and Raytheon,[1] two of the major missile manufacturers and defense contractors, unhappy with their image as warmakers, have moved into a popular and profitable new business. With the aid of community psychiatrists, these corporations are making special teaching films and programmed learning devices aimed at dissuading high school students from taking drugs. The films emphasize the establishment's ideology that drugs lead to the ruin of reputation, career, and property. Community psychiatrists are thus providing the linkages between the military-industrial complex and the medical-industrial complex.[14]

5. *The Military.* More direct links with the military are demonstrated by psychiatrists[23] who have helped soldiers and officers deal with their anxiety about killing and being killed in Viet Nam.[24] In effect, the Army utilizes community mental health to make its men into a more efficient and brutal killing machine.

Other community psychiatrists aid American imperialism by working with the CIA.[26]

6. *Morals.* Psychiatrists and other therapists have been defining and defending the morals of the system. For example, psychiatrists have encouraged monogamy, male supremacy, and heterosexuality, at the same time labeling everything else as "deviant." Whether the psychiatrist admits it or not, at every point in the therapeutic program, whether in his office or the community, he prescribes a set of values which in turn describe and support the establishment's moral-political judgments and values.[12]

Community psychiatry not only supports the prevailing politics and mores, but also it utilizes a repressive ideology to destroy dissident politics and mores. For example, a few radical students will "trash" a building. The radicals' politics will be transformed into psychopathology and their Oedipal complexes will be carefully examined in scores of scholarly papers.[2] On the other hand, President Nixon can reach historic levels of bombing and violence in Viet Nam and no community psychiatrist is consulted on the President's Oedipal complex or psychopathology.

Whether it be the "neurotic" housewife, "acting out" pupils or "paranoid" student radicals, community psychiatry has become a central ideological instrument for obscuring people's understanding of their experience and for preventing them from recognizing the social bases and collective nature of their oppression. The basic mechanism by which community psychiatry achieves this is to reduce all collective experience to a sum of individual experiences, to reduce all social grievances to individual pathology. Racism and sexism, exploitation and imperialism disappear, save as triggers of latent psychopathology. Conceived of in scholarly journals, boiled down by pop psychiatrists, advice columnists, and consultants, community psychiatry has become the pseudoscientific underpinning for a repressive ideology which promotes alienation from oneself, from others, and from reality.

In terms of community mental health services and programs it must be noted that programmatic decisions are made on virtually a totally materialistic basis. The "success," "failure," or survival of a particular mental health service has little or nothing to do with its health-enhancing qualities or therapeutic efficacy. Survival of a program is primarily determined by whether or not the program or service enhances or protects its parent system or that system's institutional, professional, and personal priorities, profits, prerogatives, and prestige. All too often the definition of "community psychiatry" as those programs which keep the community safe for psychiatrists has become the reality of community mental health programs. Too many psychiatrists and community mental health specialists seem to believe that the primary purpose of mental health programs is to prevent, rather than to foment, social action. As one past president of the American Psychiatric Association said: "Administrators and deliverers of mental health services will have to sharpen their perception and recognition of their responsibilities *in maintaining social homeostasis.* They bear a social responsibility much in the *same way as the courts and other law enforcement agencies do.*" (Emphasis added, R. K.)

The political value (i.e., value to the system) of a mental health program helps determine and define its success or failure. One example is the role of the community mental health center as a pacification program, particularly as "law and order" issues become more visible and viable, and it becomes politically more profitable to "keep down the natives." As J. M. Statman[22] points out, pacification produced by the use of massive armed force ". . . represents only one and not necessarily the most effective means of inducing obedience." It is often the employment of only minimal force ". . . which proves to be the most effective. This may be especially true if such force is presented in a form which is not readily perceived as coercive or which, in fact, is seen as helpful in intent by both the agents of oppression and the oppressed. The mystification of experience which accompanies the acceptance of such 'kindness' creates a form of oppression far more destructive than that of the armed occupier." Thus, in the urban ghetto and elsewhere, "it is the social worker, the psychologist, the educator and the community psychiatrist who play the key oppressive roles, who have become the 'soft police'."

Community mental health programs, in general, do serve to pacify a neighborhood, particularly a ghetto, and thus are functionally racist. The community mental health programs ". . . mystify and mollify justifiable outrage and thereby prevent action for meaningful change." By directing community concern toward problems of "mental health" and away from "efforts to confront the basic oppressive institutions in our society, such programs function to maintain the establishment's status quo, rather than to advance the interests of the oppressed community."

It thus appears that community mental health programs divert community energies from more meaningful efforts, that they depoliticize issues and instead "psychiatricize" issues, that the employment of community leaders co-opts them and alienates them from their community and "thereby weakens the community power base," and that such programs, no matter how good their intentions may be, can not turn against their funding source and one of the community's major oppressing agents—the government.

2. The U. S. Politico-economic System as the Major Cause of Psychiatric Disability

Unless one accepts a genetic factor and/or a "downward drift" factor as the primary cause(s) of mental problems, all mental illness is derived from a social matrix which is always determined by the institutions which legitimize power and economic relationships among the classes[18], races, and sexes of that society.[10] It is these institutions which must be altered if we are to mount a serious attack against mental illness.

If psychiatry serves the system and the system in turn causes mental disability, what is the community psychiatrist to do, and more importantly what is the community to do? For the community psychiatrist to practice in a conventional way in contemporary American society, especially in ghetto areas, is about as corrupt as being a practicing community psychiatrist in a concentration camp. While we do not yet live in concentration camp conditions, we are not all that far from it to disregard the connections. Even if the psychiatrist provides services in the concentration camp, even if he really meets some people's needs in the camp and is supportive to them, the psychiatrist in such a political environment can function only as a part of a pacification program within the camp and thus support the concentration camp, working counter to the prisoner's most crucial and urgent needs, i.e., getting out of and causing the destruction of the camp. The concentration camp psychiatrist, if he chooses to function in the camp in his customary way, will have as his first priority the meeting of personal and professional needs, i.e., he will function as a traditional psychiatrist, regardless of the political and social setting and regardless of the people's need to destroy the camp. Thus, to meet his personal and professional needs first is to function in a totally corrupt fashion. The only responsible, socially utilitarian way he can function is to be a politico-military organizer or technician—all in the service of the destruction of the camp.[13] The community psychiatrist in the camp, giving traditional services, can function only to adjust the patient or prisoner to the concentration camp or ghetto. Services provided, no matter how technologically innnovative and advanced, are of no value unless they help destroy the conditions that are destroying the community. At least in real concentration camps, most people know what they are in, because they came there from the outside and they recognize the disparity between their former and present lives. The higher the visibility of this disparity, the greater the degree of heightened political consciousness produced, and the greater their ease in dealing with the situation.

COMMUNITY CONTROL OF COMMUNITY MENTAL HEALTH

Community control must be seen in its broadest sense, namely that in which a community itself controls and determines the political, social, and economic realities of the community. We cannot talk about community mental health without a community and we cannot talk about a community until it has a political consciousness of itself and is self-controlled. The fight for and the achievement of real control of the community, by and for the community, will ultimately determine just how therapeutic our communities can be.

In terms of community controlled community mental health services, psychiatrists in the community will not be allowed to practice in their customary fashion. A community controlled community will attempt to integrate all services into a human services network, including community controlled schools, fire departments, and police.[25] The community seeks to control these services to eliminate professional and institutional priorities and biases.

One example of professional, establishment, and institutional imperatives holding sway over community need is the addiction crisis. Community psychiatrists and other community mental health specialists view addiction as a personality problem and talk of the so-called "addictive personality." However, there is a far greater correlation between addiction and economic and geographic distribution than with personality types. Yet, treatment programs are geared for changing individual personalities and not the political realities which are responsible for the addiction problems. The immediate political realities are the Mafia, police complicity, and political payoffs throughout the city. Professor R. Cloward of Columbia University notes that political inaction on the part of the government existed and the narcotics traffic tolerated as long as the inaction and tolerance aided the establishment's status quo. "As long as slum dwellers remain on drugs they cannot mobilize politically," said Cloward. The Black Panthers prohibit the use of narcotics for just that reason.[19] In the face of the above, no existing drug treatment program so far has been shown to be a serious and efficacious one, and none relates to political realities. The only one which does is that of the People's Defense Leagues. The people of these organizations know that the political system kills one hundred addicts per month in New York City alone.[8] Thus, the violence is already there and the question of whether or not the Leagues' response should be violent is academic. The People's Defense Leagues function as vigilante groups, shooting and killing major drug pushers on sight. The Leagues are having more therapeutic effect on the community in general, and the addicts in particular, than any extant treatment program. And to be sure, no community psychiatrist ever thought of such a program or researched its possibilities, but people from the community did.

How can community control of mental health services be seriously effective if the community has no understanding of community psychiatry? Community control refers to the community's controlling the over-all policies and priorities of the services. The community, through its elected board, would make decisions about, for example, whether the treatment program should have a long-term, individual, psychoanalytic orientation or, for example, whether addiction services should be emphasized, or whether research and training programs should be emphasized over direct services. The community not only has a right to control its service, (after all, as a minimum rationalization for community control, services for mental health are well over fifty percent publicly funded and thus should be publicly controlled) but also has a necessity and an ability to make decisions relevant to itself. It might require an "expert" to determine the relative harm of the side-effects of Mellaril versus Thorazine, but a community can evaluate the over all relevance of various services offered.

Is there a danger in giving the "layman" too much say? The danger is not in giving him (her), i.e., the community, enough say. Without community control, services and professionals are accountable to no one, priorities are determined privately and secretly, and artificial hierarchies are maintained. More dangerous than not giving the community what it deserves is the community's failure to demand and take what is its own. The professional's attempts to deny the community its rights of self-determination, with the rationalization that the community may not be familiar with certain techniques and technology, is akin to former President Johnson's ignoring the public's criticism of the Viet Nam war because ". . . the public doesn't have all the facts." It has not been necessary to be a general in My Lai to know that the U. S. has no legitimate business in Viet Nam. By the same token, one does not have to be a psychiatrist to understand that long-term, individual, psychoanalytic therapy has little relevance to a community at large.

What will community control do about professionalism? Professionalism encourages artificial hierarchies, as well as manpower and womanpower shortages. The professional earns more than the worker. The fight for deprofessionalization does not mean that everyone winds up with the same extent of knowledge and skills. We will always need a division of labor, where some technicians have some special expertise. But possession of expertise, according to the community, in no way should legitimize power to set policy and maintain privilege, such as higher salaries.

Nobody is suggesting that there be no standards set, say, for surgeons. What the community is saying and demanding is that those standards not be arbitrary and exclusionary, that they be based on fact and function and not privilege, that they be open to public scrutiny and review, and that there be different routes by which one achieves those standards, e.g., academic training versus on-the-job training with open-ended career ladders.

The ideal professional works to put his profession out of business. For example, a doctor's ultimate goal should be to end all sickness and disability, so that the medical profession is no longer needed.

Is not the mental health profession already working towards many of the goals sought by the community in its demand for community control? For example, if a universal or national health insurance plan was enacted would it not remove some of the class, race, and sex distinctions of psychiatric services? National health insurance might allow for more people to afford individual, private psychotherapy, but not many more, given the severe shortages and maldistribution of therapists. The real issues of class, race, and sex distinctions would not and could not be dealt with as long as there remain class, race, and sex distinctions in the society at large. Integrating a person psychologically or socially is integrating him (her) into a racist, sexist society. The more so-called mental health services do this, the more they serve the system which destroys the community.

Individual "patients" acting alone, even with the financial resources of a national health insurance plan, cannot organize services or demand services that are politically relevant and personally responsive. Only groups of people and communities can do that.

Only the community, by controlling its own services, can insure that those services serve the community. The recipients of the services, therefore, must have ultimate say as to the shape, form, and function of those services. Those served must be able to have the same modes of communication and contacts as does the so-called professional. For example, professional journals must be people's journals. Theory and practice must come from the bottom-up and not top-down. Practice and service must be totally accountable to those receiving the services. The degree to which services are not totally accountable is the degree to which those services are a tool of pacification. Without community control the profession guarantees that it will continue to perpetuate staff shortages and monopolization of technology, and that what quality services exist will only go to those with the financial resources to get them.

Community mental health training programs must be drastically altered and control of these programs removed from psychiatrists. The facts[16] are that most so-called well-trained psychiatrists, that is, those trained at our best university institutions, have a limited understanding of how the human personality functions because their knowledge is based almost exclusively on a Freudian understanding of personality development, to the neglect of entire areas of knowledge in psychology, sociology, anthropology, economics, and political science.[27]

Community control would prevent the gerrymandering of catchment areas to suit the upper middle class needs of psychiatric institutions.[7] The purpose of catchment areas was to prevent the arbitrary exclusion of patients from treatment centers and to insure that all clients within a catchment area received the same care from publicly funded institutions—in other words, to protect the community. Institutional opposition to catchment areas stems from the recognition that communities will define catchment areas and not private institutions. Publicly and politically defined cathment areas divide the community along lines of rational needs, as opposed to lines of institutional empire and exploitation.

In practical terms, institutional opposition to catchment areas arises from the vision of community controlled funding, planning, and administration for entire catchment areas. Imperialistically oriented professionals shrink from the day, which is rapidly approaching, where a "lay" board of catchment area residents will write contracts for services from professional institutions and then will evaluate the services rendered. Will the community be fascinated by the profession's precious research projects? Will they be glad to hear how many Park Avenue psychiatrists they have funded through training? Will the profession be ready to face people sitting across a table from them, rather than lying passively on beds and couches?

Perhaps the most threatening aspect of catchment areas is that they *define institutional responsibility.* Given a catchment area, an elite, so-called private institution is assigned a community which it must relate to, a public that it must account to. Geographic assignments ultimately threaten the institution's "right" to select its patients (an extrapolation of the psychiatrist's "right" to select interesting, wealthy patients). But the mental health profession's uneasiness about geographic responsibility may stem from an even deeper fear, the fear that its institutions could not fulfill this responsibility, even if it could *accept* it. Psychiatric institutions really have very little to offer a community that is demanding mental *health* services, as opposed to mental illness "removal." The catchment area that is lucky enough to gain a conventional community mental health center in its bounds may soon discover that the emperor has no clothes—or worse—the wrong politics.

REFERENCES

1. Berson, G., Corporate bummer, *Hard Times,* Mar. 16, 1970, p. 2.
2. Burlage, R., The medical means of repression, *Health PAC Bulletin,* May, 1970, p. 2.
3. Fishbein, M., Psychiatry and the future, *Medical World News,* Mar. 17, 1969, p. 62.
4. Ginzberg, E., *Men, Money and Medicine,* Columbia University Press, New York, 1969, p. 24.
5. Kenny, M., Cops: from clubs to couches, *Health PAC Bulletin,* May, 1970, pp. 11-13.
6. Kenny, M., Mental health outposts: winning the hearts and minds, *Health PAC Bulletin,* May, 1969, pp. 8-10.
7. Kenny, M., Up against the mental bloc, *Health PAC Bulletin,* Dec., 1969, pp. 4-10.
8. Kunnes, R., Community control of community health, *The New Physician,* Jan., 1970, pp. 28-33.
9. Kunnes, R., How to be a radical therapist, *The Radical Therapist,* April, 1971, (in press).
10. Kunnes, R., Politics and psychiatry, *Interface,* Vol. 3, No. 3, Feb., 1971, pp. 5-7.

Radicalism and Community Mental Health   49

11. Kunnes, R., Psychiatry: instrument of the ruling class, *The Radical Therapist*, April, 1970, pp. 4-6.
12. Kunnes, R., Repression: psychiatry as an agent of the establishment, *McGill Medical Journal*, Oct., 1970, pp. 68-72.
13. Kunnes, R., Seizure of services: a case study of health expropriation, *McGill Medical Journal*, Oct., 1969, pp. 6-8.
14. Kunnes, R., *Your Money Or Your Life: The Medical Market Place*, Dodd, Mead & Co. New York, 1972, pp. 150-155.
15. Kunnes, R., The U. S. health delivery system: a brief politico-economic analysis, *McGill Medical Journal*, Oct., 1969, pp. 99-101.
16. Kunnes, R., Will the real community psychiatry please stand up, *International Journal of Psychiatry*, Vol. 9, pp. 304-305.
17. Locke, K., Therapy is political change . . . not peanut butter, *The Radical Therapist*, Oct., 1970, p. 1.
18. Miller, S. M., and E. Mishler, Social class, mental illness and American psychiatry, *Milbank Memorial Fund Quarterly*, April, 1959, pp., 174-190.
19. *New York Times,* March 19, 1970, p. 29.
20. Ochberg, F., and E. Trickett, Administrative responses to racial conflict in high school, *Community Mental Health Journal*, Dec., 1970, pp. 470-475.
21. Rainwater, L., and W. L. Yancy, *The Moynihan Report and the Politics of Controversy*, MIT Press, Cambridge, 1967, pp. 474-478.
22. Statman, J., Community mental health as a pacification program, *American Journal of Orthopsychiatry*, Mar., 1970, p. 274.
23. Talbot, J., Community psychiatry in the army, *Journal of the American Medical Association*, Vol. 210, No. 7, pp. 1233-1237.
24. Tiffany, W., Army psychiatry in the mid-sixties, *American Journal of Psychiatry*, Vol. 123, No. 8, 1967, p. 819.
25. Waskow, A., Community control of the Police, *Trans-action*, Dec., 1969, pp. 4-7.
26. Wedge, B., Khrushchev at a distance, *Trans-action*, Vol. 5, No. 10, 1968, pp. 24-28.
27. Werry, J., On psychiatric imperialism, *The Radical Therapist*, Nov., 1970, p. 5.

AGAINST THE RADICAL POSITION IN COMMUNITY MENTAL HEALTH

Lawrence C. Kolb

My understanding of the meaning of the community mental health movement in the United States generates from the Community Mental Health Act passed in 1963 during the Kennedy administration. There were two major parts to that act, first, a new form of delivery of service within the community and, second, education of the public and prevention. In regard to delivery of service, funding has been arranged for the establishment of health centers or a network of health centers in areas where the distribution was poor. This would make it possible for people who had been receiving inadequate services through the media of large state hospitals to be treated much nearer to their homes so that there could be early diagnosis. At the same time, they would be near to their families so that the network of social relations need not be broken. They would be nearer their jobs, their vocations and avocations, so that the potential for reestablishment in the community would be enhanced. And they would be near their friends and other supports so that these mechanisms which sustain health and acceptance would remain intact.

I think the City of New York is a classic example of how we are tied up with a delivery system of mental health (as a matter of fact, of all health) which is antiquated. We have two large receiving hospitals and then we have a series of rather remote hospitals taking care of those who remain ill more than several weeks. In spite of the new efforts of general hospital operations, these are too few and scattered. In order to improve the services to

51

people in this vast metropolitan area we would need a wide distribution of community mental health centers to take care of the primary problems in the correction of illness. That is, we would need the establishment in local areas of clinics and clinic hospital operations in which we would provide immediate diagnosis and treatment near home. I am convinced the operation of community mental health centers of these kinds would greatly reduce the chronic hospitalism which occurs if people are sent away to institutions with the kinds of serious mental health problems or illnesses that we service. As a matter of fact, studies done by this department and other hospital groups in this city already illustrate this. Whereas the delivery system established by the City and State of New York will transfer forty percent of the patients from the big centers of Bellevue and Kings County Hospitals, when you have a community mental health center dealing with a local area you will very quickly find that professionals working in such an area will reduce transfers to the remote chronic hospitals to about ten percent.

I am very dedicated to this aspect of the community mental health program. When it comes to the other aspects of the program—education and prevention—here I believe there has been a tremendous amount of loose thinking and we have become confused.

In the matter of prevention, perhaps our friends in public health did not help the situation by drawing all kinds of activities of medical and mental health people under the wing of prevention. All treatment is now tertiary prevention and rehabilitation is now secondary prevention. When they talk about primary prevention in the area of psychiatry the possibilities are very limited indeed. They may involve the rare metabolic disturbances that lead to mental deficiencies or conditions such as Wilson's disease, but I know of no primary prevention technique today to take care of the major problems such as schizophrenia, the psychosis of the aged, the manic-depressive psychosis, the psychoneurosis, or the psychophysiologic disturbances. The vast majority of these conditions are beyond the potential of any primary preventive measure. On the other hand, I agree with many others that early detection and treatment will sustain many of these people in the community, maintain their health, and contribute to the general social welfare.

The community mental health center would reach large masses of people in communities where people are willing to accept it. I believe this to be highly desirable and in communities with such mental health centers many have received early diagnosis and therapy who would not do so before. However, I have serious doubts that such a mental health center can be placed in every community. In fact, it seems that the very communities that need them the most, that is, the central city ghetto areas, are the least well educated and the least accepting. Our social science studies done here indicate that in the most crowded and impoverished areas, where the people are most deprived, they are the least accepting of mental illness. In fact, they would like to see the seriously ill removed to a remote hospital. The large hospital at a distance is seen as an asylum by those in the overcrowded ghetto. Yet the original professional aim of the Community Mental Health Act is the correct one and a teaching program that might change this attitude would be very useful. Even so, it would seem that there would have to be radical changes in the nature of the living conditions of the masses in the ghetto. Education alone cannot do it. There would also have to be more space, more jobs, and more recreational facilities before these people are liable to take the liberal positions that one finds in individuals living in the less crowded and more affluent urban and suburban areas.

The rate of development of the community mental health center is a matter of concern to the radicals who feel that one must do everything immediately. From what I have just said, which comes from well-established studies done by competent social scientists, it is clear that pushing the notion down the throats of ghetto area people that they should have a mental health center to take care of people near home is just as autocratic a position and as lacking in compassion as the positions of those who have been in charge of programs in the past. The radicals suffer from a certain elitism too in their proposed dedication to individuals in the deprived areas. It is my belief that one may not impose the opinions of a few persons on a community, whether they happen to be identified as radicals or conservatives in the field of mental health.

There are individuals who feel that only if the mental health centers are engaged in political activities will the aims of these centers be achieved. Here I would state categorically that they thus identify themselves as being ahistoric. We have right now the fifty-year experience of the effectiveness of similar theories applied in a very great country, the USSR. We also have the experience of those countries in the English-speaking world that have adopted programs of socialized medicine. Let us start with Russia. Here it was thought that by establishing political activity that applied to all the people in the state and with educational plans deriving from that political theory providing a presumed equality, it would be possible to eradicate mental illness. Well, it simply has not happened. Russian psychiatrists thought when the program went through that by making it possible to develop their population to the highest level of socialized man, all mental illness would disappear. They now frankly admit that no change whatsoever has occurred in the incidence or prevalence of such a serious problem as schizophrenia and they admit that this is as great a problem for them as it is for the rest of the world. They still seek to determine whether they have either prevented or reduced the incidence and prevalence of neurosis and personality disturbance. Reports from Russia show that they have problems of drug abuse. Their alcoholism problem is immense. They are having problems with their young people. It is obviously impossible to establish exact equivalences between the discovering, identifying, and reporting methods of various countries. For example, we had thought from the reports from the USSR that there was a reduction in beds needed for psychiatric care in that country. However, this was largely due to the absence of older people in

their mental hospitals. It turned out that in their bureaucracy the elderly are not seen by psychiatrists but are
taken care of by the Department of Social Welfare. In
short, this great social experience which grows out of a
very radical political movement has failed to demonstrate that it has made any dent in the incidence or prevalence of the serious mental illnesses and there is equally
great doubt that it affects what we commonly recognize
as psychoneuroses, psychosomatic illness, and so forth.

If you look at the figures from England, New Zealand,
and Australia you will find much the same. The same
problems that confront American psychiatrists and
those in other mental health disciplines in this country
confront their people. They perhaps provide better distributed services than we do, but on the other hand it is my
belief that they are short on manpower and they do not
provide the quality for certain segments of the population that we do.

In the matter of community control, here the radicals
say that the spoken voice of a local community will
provide better services in a particular area than the
operation of a professional administration, the support
of a Board of Trustees, and a medical advisory board
selected from professional staff. It seems to me that the
time has gone when voluntary hospitals will appoint to
their Boards only people from the population at large
rather than assuring themselves of contributions of
people from the local communities served by the institutions. There must be representation of the local community. Now the problem as I see it, as posed by the
radicals and those in the government who seem to be
convinced that there should be a controlling local board
is as follows: There has not been a single directive from
any federal or state agency willing to define the nature of
representation. Nor have I heard a single community
leader, corporation leader, or elected representative
stand and define it. It has surprised me that all of these
groups, while speaking of community control, have been
quite unwilling to define how one gets a representative
group from a community.

As a matter of fact, when one looks at the radicals

advocating community control who participate in many meetings, one finds that few have lived in the community, and instead they have appeared on the scene propelled by some inner drive, which one cannot determine but which allows them to state their dedication to the people of the community.

I have made the proposition that a service which is to be available to a local catchment area, as it is called, and which provides for a community board, should be assured representation from every health area in that community. In that way it is more likely to reflect the various ethnic groups living in different parts of the community. For instance, in northern Manhattan we have a community which consists of first- and second-generation citizens who came from Germany immediately before or after World War II. We also have a vast first-, second-, and third-generation group of Irish Catholics. We have a growing population of blacks, some of whom have just arrived from the South. We have a group from Puerto Rico and there are smaller groups of Greek and Chinese descent. The local community group here has not sought representation from all of the ethnic groups in this very complex community. It seems to me a real need to have representation from each of the health areas served.

I would think that such a board should have both lay and professional representation. And when it comes to the professional representation I would not subscribe to limiting this to mental health professionals; any of the major professions could be included since there are many which have been concerned with the human problems falling under the scope and responsibility of those in the mental health professions.

In one of the early community meetings I attended there was a vote taken by the group to remove from the so-called Council of the time all those persons who were not living in the community. I think they were right to a certain extent, but there is also a weakness in this position. No community is filled with all the wisdom in the world and any community which wants quality care will want to seek advice from professionals and nonprofessionals outside the community. Any community board should have a series of places open for capable persons outside the community to maintain and control the quality of their service.

So I feel that representation on a community board should be defined as representation from each of the health areas within a health district and, in addition, that there must be professionals on the board. As I have already said, there is very little that we may be able to do in regard to prevention, so to provide able treatment we must have those on the board who have the knowledge and skills and regard their voice as an important one.

In my opinion, most of the pressure for community control comes from groups who really wish to ascertain that those they represent, particularly the minority groups, have a potential for appointment to the significant offices of the center and have a potential for employment in the local center. I think their dedication should also be to the potential for finding the proper people to take care of those in the community who are ill. Those community mental health centers which establish boards dedicated to job-seeking goals will assuredly never have a first-class staff. They will assuredly deprive the people of that area of the kinds of assistance they would wish to give to members of their own family. I have been struck that when radicals who insist on community control become ill themselves or have a family member or a friend ill, they quickly find a way to obtain the assistance of those professional groups working in a well-established institution who are known to be competent. Able staff, both professional and nonprofessional, tend to fix themselves to institutions where there is some recognition of their potential. In other words, when it comes to dealing with matters of the soul or body, there is no doubt that most people like to receive their sustenance from those who are properly trained to manage their affairs. If the community mental health center is to be dedicated to the prevention and care of mental illness, then it should not be a social welfare station or political club.

It would seem that, if the community has strong feelings about it, the arrangement of the board could be such as I believe has been set up at Boston University. There, lay persons are appointed to the board and are given a controlling voice in the final appointment of an individual to a senior position as well as a conspicuous voice in personnel matters. However, for good administration, the administrator, once appointed, should certainly have a sufficient amount of freedom to pursue the programs he feels are important. The senior positions, the administrative positions must be filled by professionals. Furthermore, community boards must recognize that in the professions, experience is of great importance. They should require that those who are appointed to the post of senior administrator or as heads of various components of these institutions are qualified by their professional organizations. This means that such individuals will have had to demonstrate their abilities through active practice and experience in one city or another over periods extending from five to ten years beyond the granting of a professional degree.

Some of those who label themselves as radicals amongst the professional groups today believe that establishing a community board will allow their views to prevail in the operation of the community mental health center and that by following a certain political line the centers will be able to facilitate change not only in the giving of health care but also in the social system. To my mind, this is another fallacy in thinking. In the United States today we have so many groups of people from so many parts of the world who have lived for differing periods of time in this country that we have a tremendous diversity of opinion. In some sections of the country there are first generations of people who have immigrated from political regimes where they discovered that the opinions of an elite socialistic group or an elite authoritarian group in their own countries were not to the benefit of all. These people would be opposed to many of the radical views (which I think are tainted with really old fashioned socialism) and they might even reject and oppose the opinions put forth by a liberal and enlightened professional management.

Another point that needs to be considered is the

problem of manpower and its relation to the rate at which effective community mental health centers can be established. Some years ago when this program was first brought forward many professors of psychiatry expressed doubt that the manpower was available to provide the staffing for these centers and they recommended caution. The manpower situation has really not improved in any of the professions related to community mental health. As a matter of fact, at present in the National Institute of Mental Health there seems to be an attempt to reduce funding for training programs. Manpower and the quality of manpower has a great deal to do with the effectiveness of provision of service. The establishment of large numbers of small centers, understaffed or partially staffed by young professionals or paraprofessionals, will hardly be able to service or to achieve the described aims of the centers. In fact, considering the distribution of these centers as presently approved by the federal agencies, it would seem that the populations most in need of them have been the least capable of applying and have not received them. And yet if these centers are placed in the deprived areas of great cities or in rural areas, their potential for getting manpower is seriously impaired. I do not believe that the filling out of a mental health center in any part of the country with a group of paraprofessionals is really going to help the mental health of the community. As a matter of fact, it is nothing more than cheating the deprived communities. People from the black and Puerto Rican communities who we see in our medical center are as interested in getting the best quality care from a well-trained person as people from any other group. Merely making large groups of jobs available to persons who have no great knowledge of the problems of stress-induced illness or the recognized mental health problems will bring little respect or little relief to these people.

In planning for community mental health centers, the radicals that I have known seem to have no interest in reviewing the extensive reports made by the regional mental health planning boards. These boards were set up shortly after the Act was passed and they spent many months studying various aspects of the need for community mental health centers, that is, the need in terms of the placement facilities, problems to be cared for, and manpower requirements. My experience with the leaders of the radical movement of the past few years indicates that they have either not read these documents at all or, if they have read them, failed to comprehend them. Also, if one requests any definitive plans or programs from the radical group, they are not available.

Here is an example from my own experience. One of the radical techniques is to use the revolutionary or labor movement tactics of confrontation. Since these people generally are a small group in a community it is necessary to arouse a considerable commotion in attacking some proposed program. If they can get the press and TV interested, they pour forth to the public many statements which distort and vilify what is going on. Thus a great fuss was made about a proposed institution in which it was stated that this institution only had two doors, one for whites and one for blacks. The facts were that the plans were drawn by the City of New York with the aid of the University and had what one would usually expect, all of the openings and entries which one would find in any hospital. Furthermore, there were plans for a series of satellite clinics, six for the area in question, with the provision for 400 health positions and an annual budget around four million dollars. Did the radicals ever read the plans? Did they ever report this to the public? No. As a matter of fact, in questioning the New York City Community Mental Health Board and the University, they asked if plans were available and when told that they were, said that they wished to read them. Two representatives came to my office and when the plans were offered they left saying they only wanted to test the integrity of the speaker. Those plans have never been read.

I might as well discuss the effectiveness of the radical movement. The people of the community I mentioned above, to whom the radicals presume to dedicate themselves, have not had a single addition to service in the three years since the movement commenced. They have not received a single new health-care job and only a very few individuals, probably less than ten, have received any new jobs. It is difficult for me to find in radical efforts of this type either dedication to their fellow man or effectiveness in tactics. They have failed to do the careful planning or make the series of moves which would really bring about the development of sound programs to help the ill and deprived in local communities.

I would have to say the same thing in regard to prevention and the idea of using political means to bring it about. We have to ask those who plan vast preventive programs to be very specific about the conditions they propose to prevent, the procedures they propose to use, and the numbers of cases that may be prevented. It is possible to ask these questions. And just as we arc asked to evaluate treatment procedures in hospitals we must also require that those who advance propositions regarding prevention also subject themselves to evaluation.

Some who support radical trends in the management of mental health centers insist there should be a major revision of the training programs. Just what the revision should be is not clear, although some say that the various institutions retain programs too long and make attacks on the individual therapy system used in many places. Once again I think we must go back to the nature of the problem confronting the mentally ill in this country. The vast majority of persons coming to mental health centers would not require prolonged hospitalization, but we may as well recognize that there is a percentage, probably less than twelve percent, who will require a considerable period of hospitalization and other treatment for their proper care. This will also require the skills of highly trained individuals, professional and nonprofessional. While community centers may not be set up to give more than two or three months of treatment, I would hope that the local center could provide the whole gamut of training. The idea that these centers would be a rapid turnover advisory center where there would be great excitement and that students would flock to such an institution seems in error to me. Students flock to those institutions where they are likely to be taught by people with experience and skill. When we are dealing with problems of human behavior and their surcease through psychotherapeutic and psychopharmacological means, the major measures of today, then we are dealing with a highly complex series of teachings. And the record of teaching institutions clearly shows that students go where they will get the best and appropriate supervision. It is true that amongst students today there will be some who will be caught up with the enthusiastic statement that there is much to be learned by attending an institution dedicated to the radical point of view. But I suspect that in that group there will be a considerable number leaving, in very short order, filled with disillusionment.

I think that the notion that all problems may be solved in a short period of time through some kind of brief technical or social engineering plan is going to be a failure and, in fact, will detract from the interest in the field. Will it be possible through the radical ideas of social engineering to materially affect mental health in our country? From the studies we have done of the population in northern Manhattan, it is apparent that the use of psychiatric hospitalization is very much higher amongst those who live in more economically deprived areas, as a matter of fact it is three times the size per 1000 population. These are also areas in which there is a lack of job opportunities, in which the school system is deteriorating, infant mortality is higher, the drug problem is severe, and delinquency and criminal activity are high. Can a group of radicals or mental health activists affect the social functioning of people in such an area? My own belief, based on observation of the people requiring the greater amount of hospitalization, is that many of them are suffering from stress syndromes, serious problems that are relieved very frequently and very rapidly following a short period of hospitalization from a week to two weeks. It might well be that if social conditions were changed there would be much less need for the hospital care of such persons. On the other hand there are theoretical positions from the field of genetics stating that individuals found in this area are genetically impaired or from the field of sociology stating that people who find themselves in these areas of the cities arrived there through the "drift hypothesis." Current data will not substantiate one point of view or another.

I personally would like to see a number of grand social experiments in which such areas of our cities were upgraded in all respects—in terms of the funding, in terms of the assurance of jobs for all which would lead to self-respect, in terms of the security for families, in terms of the needed space for living and for recreational areas. But can this be done through a group of professionals working in a series of small mental health centers? I would seriously doubt this. We operate with a two party political system. The professional might well be able to organize these communities to support one political party or the other, but once one identifies with one party it is unlikely that one would receive support from the other. The best position for the professional is to give advice as to the needs of the community and relate to both parties. Attempting to establish an independent party amongst a limited number of deprived communities in this country has never been very successful. In short, it is very likely that the politically active radical therapist in the community mental health center will do more harm to the movement than good. He is likely to offend those in the on-going government bureaus and may very well end up removing from our support that which we have obtained with so much difficulty in this past quarter of a century.

It seems to me that the proper position of the professional in this field is as a spokesman and advisor to the communities in which they work; a professional advisor to those who are responsible for political representation at the city, state, or federal level. Here the professional achieves a degree of respect since he is known to be knowledgeable and presumably would be able to provide to the practitioners of politics the kinds of information they would need to foster the welfare of the people they represent. When the professional appears on the scene as an active politician he will probably come to realize, after some time, that he is an extraordinary novice. Politics, too, is a profession which one has to learn over a long period of time. It requires the development of a sound and stable network as well. The representation that many of those in the radical mental health movement have made will, I doubt, be very impressive amongst those serving the various political views in this country. Once again a naive or gauche appearance of a mental health professional on the political scene will not, in the long run, serve the purposes to which he believes he has dedicated himself.

What is the future of the community mental health center? I see it really as a community hospital with outreaches of one kind or another into the community. These outreaches would be a series of satellite clinics in areas where one can do case finding and where people of different backgrounds can gather and present themselves. In terms of the future of the community mental health movement, it seems to me that there is a growing realization amongst those who are concerned with the development of future policies and plans regarding health in general that the various segments of the health scheme cannot be effectively managed separately. In the future development of community mental health centers more attention must be paid to relating them to the development of general health centers. I believe that the movement away from medicine, which has been suggested by some, is a grave mistake. The dedication of medicine to the care of the sick in this country is very great and it will continue. The potential of achieving a different kind of support under another term, such as mental health, is not likely to obtain the backing of large numbers in the community or from those who will be deciding priorities with funding. Many in the mental health disciplines fail to recognize that they have yet to be accepted by the public at large and that many times their presence is looked upon with doubt or suspicion. This is particularly true of those who know our country less well or who are not well educated;

they are apt to consider the presence of a psychiatrist or a psychiatric social worker, or nurse or psychologist, as an insult or another form of downgrading by the establishment. For instance, we have discovered that the use of the public health nurse for community outreach work is much more accepted by the community than the use of, say, a psychiatric social worker. I understand that this has been the experience of other groups when outreach is taken under the cover of the indirect relationship with a medical group. I bring this up here as a means of indicating the necessity for increasing the relationship with general medical programs rather than separating them and presenting the mental health movement to the community as a separate entity. As a separate entity the mental health movement will have very little strength to reach the goals which many hold, including those who speak from radical positions, and will be more likely to fail than if they remain under the banner of a professional group which long since achieved an immense emotional solidarity with the public.

I would like to add to what I have stated that I believe that the community mental health movement has been the most important step taken by this country and our professional group in the last decade. Much benefit has already come from it. It has stimulated the trials of new ways of providing services. It has demonstrated that many people can be sustained near their homes. The comments which have preceded are intended to bring those who espouse the radical cause to examine whether their strategies and tactics will, in the long run, support or expand the gains which have already been achieved or if they are likely to be destructive. I would be much distressed if we should find that the great support brought about by the efforts of so many over these past several decades is lost by the hasty and thoughtless acts of a few within the next decade.

Part III
Traditional Psychotherapy

TRADITIONAL PSYCHOTHERAPY

"Traditional Psychotherapy" implies a classical model of psychotherapy. Services are professionalized and emphasis is on individual psychotherapy and long-term treatment with a psychoanalytic theoretical base. Leadership is psychiatric. Private practice is considered an ideal and the attempt is made to keep as much as possible of the qualities of private practice in a hospital or agency setting. Paralleling the tendency in private practice for responsibility to be concentrated in the hands of one therapist, the agency trys to avoid sharing clinical responsibility for patients with other agencies. Those who favor traditional psychotherapy believe that under very serious circumstances treatment should be mandated.

One group of opponents of "Traditional Psychotherapy" are antagonistic because they feel that these methods are generally not effective—in private practice or community mental health. They believe that these expensive, time-consuming procedures have not proven their worth anywhere. They assert that as many patients are likely to recover spontaneously as do through long-term individual psychotherapy or psychoanalysis. Some of these opponents may have a substitute of their own which they believe is effective, such as encounter groups or behavior therapy.

Another group of people who feel negatively on this issue are those who believe that "Traditional Psychotherapy" is effective in individual private practice or for small private clinics but, when responsibility is taken by community mental health for large masses of people, that the centers cannot afford the luxury of these procedures. Successfully treating relatively few people through long-term individual psychotherapy will mean that the large mass of people who need help will go untreated. The emphasis must be on short-term, economical, and nontraditional treatment modalities that will reach more people.

Dr. Lawrence C. Kubie, at 76, has not mellowed into a subdued role as elder statesman in the mental health field. He continued to actively explore developments in mental health and is sharply critical of what he considers bad policies or practices. Community mental health, which evokes enthusiastic praise or platitudes by most authors in the field, has met some withering criticism from Dr. Kubie. In the following article, "The Retreat from Patients," Dr. Kubie deplores some of the new trends that lead away from individual clinical work with patients and defends the value of long-term, intensive, psychoanalytic psychotherapy.

Dr. H. J. Eysenck won an international reputation for his critical research review of the effectiveness of psychoanalytic and other psychotherapeutic methods. In the article that follows, "New Approaches to Mental Illness: The Failure of a Tradition," Dr. Eysenck reviews the evidence and again concludes that traditional forms of psychotherapy are not effective. He offers as a substitute behavior therapy and indicates that the research evidence supports its claims.

THE RETREAT FROM PATIENTS: AN UNANTICIPATED PENALTY OF THE FULL-TIME SYSTEM*

Lawrence S. Kubie

The currently prevalent retreat from patients has many roots: work with patients is painful; a general tendency to undervalue clinical skills; a general failure to realize how long it takes to acquire clinical maturity; the emphasis on research for tomorrow's medicine, at the expense of service for today's needs; propaganda for service to "the community" as though this did not require the highest degree of knowledge of individual human needs; higher academic rewards (rank, status, salaries) for everything but clinical skills; the tendency of top-rank full-time professors to set a bad example by their full-time absences. Consequently, although everything to which these fugitives from patients flee is good, the results of their flight are disastrous for American medicine. In no discipline is this trend as destructive or as prevalent as in psychiatry.

In private conversations the late Dr. Alan Gregg often used to express his concern about the penalties from which medical education might ultimately suffer because of the full-time system, of which he was a firm advocate nonetheless. He would admit that there is always a price to be paid for anything valuable, but would insist that this challenges us to discover ways of reducing this price below destructive levels. He worried

* Reprinted from *Archives of General Psychiatry*, Vol. 24, Feb. 1971, pp. 98-106, with permission of author and editor.

about the damage done by the subtle down-grading of clinical skills and clinical maturity which tends to occur under the full-time system. He would deplore the fact that in medical schools the preclinical scientist so often plays a dominant role on committees which determine policy. He attributed this to the fact that they are less heavily burdened than are the clinical teachers, who not only have to teach and do research but must also practice and furnish examples of how to take care of patients and their families at a leisurely pace. He pointed out that no matter how strictly the clinical teacher adhered to the full-time system, this responsibility of the physician to the patient and his family was vital for clinical practice and could not be hurried. Consequently, Gregg would point out, any impatience to get back to the laboratory, no matter how natural it may be, impairs the quality of this essential element in medical practice, ie, the art of being a medical naturalist, through the slow and careful and conscientious taking of medical histories.

These concerns apply to every aspect of medicine, but naturally my own concern is primarily with their significance for psychiatric education, training, and procedures. All of this is in my mind as I approach the problems which I will explore in this paper.

Whenever he tackled an unpopular topic Alan Gregg used to say, "If you are going to argue something that people do *not* want to believe, begin by indicating simply and clearly what you do *not* mean. Otherwise this is precisely what they will hear. Furthermore you will have to repeat all of this several times before they will take it in." "Only then," he would add, "can you go on to say what you *do* mean." Influenced by the sage advice of this elder statesman, I will point out that I am *not* going to say that intensive, prolonged, individual psychoanalytic psychotherapy in the setting of private practice is the only way of treating a patient, or that it is the only way of becoming a psychiatrist. What I will say is that this specific experience is one of the basic ingredients in the process of psychological exploration, and that experience of this nature is indispensable for becoming a mature psychiatrist. Note again that I do not say that it is indispensable for learning *about* psychiatry from a safe distance, but quite precisely that it is indispensable for becoming a psychiatrist. The difference between learning about and "becoming" is basic.

I also want it clearly understood that my purpose in this paper is not to belittle psychiatric research, teaching, or administration, the applications of psychiatry to our overwhelming social problems, the dedication of whole lives to these goals, or the values of group and family therapies. My purpose is rather to combat a current tendency to encourage beginners to pursue these techniques before they have had time to become psychiatrists, in fact almost as an escape from and as a substitute for the slower and more pain-filled process of "becoming."

Because I myself retired from practice, one autobiographical note is needed if I am to avoid a misunderstanding of my purpose. From time to time the need for a fresh perspective on one's self, one's life, and one's work makes it necessary to stand off at a distance from everything one has been doing. This is why I retired from practice in July 1959, but only after 30 odd years of intensive experience in psychoanalytic psychotherapy. I had been contemplating this move for more than ten years, weighing carefully its advisability, its form, and its timing. When at length I took the step, my purpose was to study, teach, and write in the setting of a psychiatric hospital. My choice of a "private" hospital was almost accidental, the result of a unique opportunity which had presented itself unexpectedly at the Sheppard and Enoch Pratt Hospital. I cannot pretend that I had foreseen the many advantages of this setting. These became clear to me only later, as I have attempted to explain in subsequent papers.[1] [2]

The move into hospital psychiatry after so many years of predominantly office practice proved to be exciting and challenging. It led me into the most fecund years of my professional life. Furthermore, the impact of this change gradually altered much of my thinking about psychiatry in general, about psychiatric training, about the formal organization of psychiatry for teaching, research, and practice, about our so-called nosology, and also about psychoanalytic theory, technique, and training. Indeed, my thinking has changed so much in these ten years that I wish that I could have 30 more years in which to subject new hypotheses to clinical test and experiemental investigation. Obviously not enough years are left to me for this—so I write and lecture about them instead. Perhaps I should have retired from private practice ten years earlier. As a matter of fact, I had tried to do so under Army auspices and had nearly succeeded when the Korean War made it impossible. Now, however, as I look back I doubt that I would have been ready at that time to take full advantage of the move. To have retired in 1949 instead of 1959 would have deprived me of many invaluable lessons learned during the final ten years of practice.

Several years ago I explored some of the factors which have always limited the rate at which it is possible for anyone to achieve maturity in psychiatry.[3] The same factors will continue to limit our rate of maturation until increasing duration of life and of mental vigor allow us more years in which to learn from mistakes. Growth in my personal understanding of the nature of the neurotic process, of its psychotic disorganization, and of the interactions with the processes of therapy did not come to me quickly. It required many years for me to free myself from intellectual bondage to the clichés which I had accepted in my earlier years in psychiatry and psychoanalysis. Others may be able to free themselves more quickly; but I learned slowly over the years by being a participant-observer of changes as these occurred in the neurotic process, sometimes spontaneously, sometimes under the influence of various combinations of therapies.

The ten years since my retirement have given me a chance to reexamine the forms of illness and of intramural and extramural therapies in relation to these varied processes of illness. (About this I again refer the reader to a series of related studies.[4,10]).

One other personal comment is relevant. The years of sober review have not turned me against my field as a

whole, nor against psychotherapy in general or psychoanalysis in particular. Instead they have shown me that
everything I have learned since retiring from practice
evolved out of the prior decades of using psychoanalysis
as a technique for the exploration of the role of the
neurotic process in human development.

Private practice has many defects, but in spite of them
it has been our best teacher for many years. There are
other ingredients, of course, and nothing that I write
here should be construed as indicating that I maintain
that there is only one way to become a psychiatrist, or
only one kind of psychiatrist to become. The psychiatrist
can and should serve many purposes for his patients, for
their families, and for society in general. What my
argument does imply is that no matter what goal any
particular student of psychiatry may envisage as his
ultimate objective, if he is to apply the lessons which
psychiatry can teach us about human life and human
society he must first become a psychiatrist. In this
process of "becoming" an indispensable ingredient will
be long and intensive personal involvement with
individual patients.

Pursued in this way, psychiatry will not be just an
abstract discipline to be studied in a classroom, in books,
in lectures, or in clinical demonstrations by others. Such
a student will become a psychiatrist by experiencing
repeatedly *within himself* the turmoil of personal growth
and change, as these are induced by repeated
experiences of interacting with and adjusting to patients
as *they* change. The process of "becoming" a psychiatrist is an experience of inner change in the psychiatrist
as changes occur in those for whose treatment he is
responsible. It is this experience which brings to us an
empathic understanding of what it means to become ill
and also to become well. Only when we lose our fear of
and our anger at psychiatric illness can we achieve this
elusive but essential combination of empathy and
objectivity which alone can enable us to identify with
sickness as well as with health. It is in this way that we
come to appreciate the universality of the neurotic
potential and of the neurotic process in its varied

disguises in all human nature.[9] Clearly my conviction that there are many ways of using psychiatry, many functions for it to perform, many roles for it to play, is not incompatible with a parallel conviction that one ingredient which is essential for *becoming* a psychiatrist as opposed to learning *about* psychiatry is the repeated experience of being a participant in the changes which occur in one's own patients over extended periods of time. (It should be self-evident that this parallels closely the process of growth in any dedicated young parent or teacher.)

To reinforce this point I will paraphrase what I have written elsewhere.[11]

Maturity as a psychiatrist is a result of the meeting of three rivers. The individual has first to work his way out of many of the conflicts which he buried in early life and which tie him to his own childhood. In one way or another (again I am not prescribing any one-and-only way) an evolving series of therapeutic experiences must occur if a man is to escape bondage to his own past in order to win his freedom to grow toward maturity as a human being. Secondly, maturity requires that he must have accepted such adult responsibilities as marriage and parenthood. It is in coping with these that he will encounter and master the problems which confront every adult as he emerges from youth. Emotional maturity of this kind is a necessary prerequisite for dealing with the problems of others from a mature basis.

Only after this can he begin to reach out for clinical maturity as a psychiatrist. Not reading, not diligent study, not psychological aptitude can supplant the experience of sustained relationships with patients as they fall ill and fall well again. Nothing can take the place of being a participant-observer of these fluctuating changes over weeks, months, and even years. Consequently the limit on the rate at which any man can achieve clinical maturity is set by the rate at which patients themselves and their illnesses can change (cf Kubie[3]).

Every young man or woman comes into this field with a starry-eyed hope not only of solving some of its

unsolved basic problems but also of being able to bring
help to many swiftly. Yet without these slow and
repeated experiences with one patient at a time, men
may acquire book-learning and may parrot what was
told to them by their elders, but they can achieve neither
personal nor professional maturity. This is why psychiatry is no field for a young man in a hurry. The young
man in a hurry will shortchange his development both
toward his own emotional maturation and toward
clinical maturity. As a consequence of hurry he will end
up incapable of mature clinical teaching, mature clinical
research, or mature clinical service.

At this point I will try to avoid another misunderstanding by pointing out that this is not in any sense a
blanket defense of psychoanalysis. I am a consistent
supporter of psychoanalysis from uninformed attacks,
but I am also its severest critic from the inside—my criticisms applying equally to the so-called orthodox and the
so-called heterodox. (Some might find it useful to read
my editorial entitled, "Missing and Wanted: A True
Heterodoxy in Psychiatry and Psychoanalysis."[12]) In
this I point out, among other things, that no scientific
discipline can grow unless it has its own built-in and un-
sparing heterodoxy, which is precisely what both psychiatry and analysis have lacked.

The Teacher as Model

Such an intensive personal involvement with patients
as I describe here is always painful. If a young resident is
to resist his natural temptation to retreat from this pain,
he will need more than the admonitions of his teachers.
He will also need their example and their moral support.
Not by precept alone but by the model which their own
professional lives hold up before their students will older
psychiatrists impress younger men with the fact that
what they stand to gain is more than worth the pain that
the process will cost. At the same time their attitudes
must show him that they appreciate the painfulness of
these struggles, that they view with sympathy and
without scorn the inevitability of the phenomena of

unconscious transference and countertransference, and that they understand the contributions which these struggles make to the learning process.

At this point I will try to avoid hurting the feelings of any friends and colleagues by introducing a disclaimer which usually is found in works of fiction: "Any resemblance to real places or persons, living or dead, is purely accidental."

Obviously no young instructor who is fresh out of his own residency can serve as an effective model, nor can an older man who early in his career turned away from work with patients. Only the clinician who kept his nose to that grindstone through many years can offer this model to younger men who show promise of future excellence but who lack maturity in clinical experience. The lack of this is a price which we are paying unexpectedly for the enormous gains which the full-time system has made possible. In all fields of medicine nonclinicians are being appointed to lead clinical departments. What is worse, young investigators from the basic sciences who are devoid of clinical experience of any kind are being appointed to posts where clinical experience is essential both for basic progress and for its human application. The reverse never occurs. Mature clinicians are never appointed to inform, guide, and criticize supposedly clinical research, although it is precisely here that mature clinical judgment is most essential.

These tendencies are further complicated by the fact that among the late-age dropouts from clinical work many turn bitterly against their earlier activities, misleading younger men into following suit. In the present stage of knowledge even the "best" psychiatrist piles up a record of mixed results: a few complete successes, many partial successes, some complete failures. The cumulative score breeds depression and anger rather than complacency. These belated angers often express the masked depressions of the older years which so often pass unrecognized, and which for many reasons occur even to successful and experienced clinicians. Why these depressions occur is a separate story; but it is well known that careeristic successes in any field give no immunity to despair.

This flight from patients is rarely a reaction to limitations which are inherent in the therapeutic processes as we know them today, grave though these are. There can be equally vivid illusions of failure after clinical successes. These illusions occur because of discrepancies between conscious and unconscious goals. A life devoted to therapy in psychiatry may lead even the skillful, experienced, and successful among us to an ill-defined sense of mourning and a weariness of the spirit. Clearly the challenge of therapy places an enormous emotional demand on all of us, whether beginners or those who after many years of experience undertake problems of increasing complexity. Yet few older psychiatrists allow themselves to think back over this, much less to talk about it. Instead they drop out in a variety of ways to be discussed below.

These dropouts are symptoms of a new disease which is inflicting itself on the corpus of psychiatry—but not of psychiatry alone, or other fields of medicine as well. It is a disease without a name whose presenting symptom is a retreat from patients not unlike the retreat of college faculties from their students, which has recently been described by Jacques Barzun.[13] The flight from patients is even better rationalized, culturally supported, and to a dismaying degree practiced, defended and approved by many eminent psychiatrists.

Where then does the dropout go? Naturally those who retreat must go some place, and usually they flee to something which is not devoid of value such as administration, which can serve many useful pruposes, community psychiatry, which has many valuable potentials for meeting human needs, research, which needs no defense, and teaching of which the same can be said. The fact remains that the flight is away from the one teacher who can continue to teach us for as long as we live, namely, the intransigent patient. Every young resident has disappointing experiences with patients with whom he has worked hard. If his professor sets before him the example of flight, the unhappy and disappointed student will be strongly tempted to imitate him. The tragic result of this will be that ultimately no one will be left in psychiatry with sufficient maturity to study his failures, much less to discover whether these failures are due to personal errors or to deficiencies which are inherent in the instrument. Psychiatry will then become what medicine would be without the clinical-pathological conference. In fact, it is on its way to this fate because under these circumstances it is natural to defend ourselves against feelings of defeat by turning on the instrument itself; especially if in so doing we again follow the example of older psychiatrists. As I consider why this is happening, I will sound like an old scold which in fact is what I am. Yet I want it to be clearly understood that I am not scolding any individual or any institution. My scolding is against a trend which has crept up on us unnoticed.

The Influence of
the Full-time System

Although this was not intended, the introduction of the full-time system into medical education unexpectedly produced in every field a tendency to place in clinical posts men who had had little or no clinical involvement with patients and who failed to understand its importance. This trend developed in psychiatry somewhat later than in other fields. In psychiatry, however, it has gathered so much momentum that in spite of the fact that psychiatry is a specially complex clinical discipline, with more variables of more different kinds than any other, today it is led primarily by men who have worked with patients only briefly or not at all, or by men who had turned away from patients as soon as they reached positions of leadership. This has obvious dangers. Even if they had had clinical experience in their earlier years, as the years pass these leaders begin to lose touch. I have been father-confessor to many. Not long ago one of them said to me, "For a long time when I was writing or teaching I could dig back into past experiences and find good clinical examples and clinical evidence. I cannot do this any more." (What others have said I will quote below.) Furthermore, out of a sense of frustration and guilt many turn against every form of psychotherapy, analytic or otherwise. Some go so far as to attack the integrity not only of the clinician who continues to do therapy but also of his patients. An obvious consequence of such attacks is the tendency of younger men to follow the example of these older men, even before the younger men have had any maturing clinical experience. Because I do not want to become involved in any *ad personam* arguments I will cite no references to specific examples of such attacks, some of which have appeared in articles in our official psychiatric journals, written by people whose names are known to all of us and whose stature is acknowledged, but who have been guilty of saying snide things in print about both patients and doctors. The more snide remarks are often directed against those patients who have any degree of financial security, as well as against their therapists. Yet these critics must know that we can learn about the role of racial, social, educational, and economic variables only by studying patients from all levels.

In some measure such attacks grow out of a misdirected decency, ie, a sincere concern among our colleagues, young and old, with our social inequities. I welcome this preoccupation of the coming generations of psychiatrists with our many unsolved social problems. Yet we must not encourage them to misuse this valid interest as an excuse for running away from the difficult and demanding task of becoming a psychiatrist. This would only convert their good-hearted purposes into the well-known pavements of a psychiatric hell.

We must also remember that many older leaders are intimidated by statistics. Unfortunately few psychiatrists (especially among the older ones) understand the pitfalls of statistics. Consequently if anyone so much as shakes a statistical stick at us, we develop butterflies in our stomachs and run for cover. If this paper succeeds in shaming us into standing ground and fighting back, we will have a chance to save the next generation from pursuing this older generation of psychiatric VIPs in their terrified flight.

Once again to avoid a misunderstanding of my

purpose I will repeat that when I deplore the indiscriminate attacks on psychotherapy, I am not defending the flaws of psychotherapy, of analysis, or of psychotherapists. Nor do I pretend that these flaws do not exist. Similarly, when I deplore the attacks on psychotherapy which so often develop out of guilt over flight, I am not maintaining that such attacks never contain any constructive and useful criticisms, no matter what mixture of conscious and unconscious biases may motivate the attacks. We know that all forms of psychiatric therapy, whether somatic or psychological or both, leave much to be desired. Yet this is not a valid reason for becoming a "dropout." For generations surgeons, internists, and pediatricians have also had to accept heartbreaking defeats. Yet they have not run away from the challenges which they have not conquered. Nor have they attacked their own field, colleagues, or patients. There must be something more than this which determines the flight of psychiatrists and their subsequent attacks on psychotherapy and therapists and patients, and especially why so many beginners run away even before they themselves have experienced defeats.

I will suggest a few explanations. Obviously a counterattack muffles the sense of guilt which most dropouts feel acutely but deny. A subtler reason is the fact already mentioned that the dropout soon begins to lose his hold on his own field. As this happens he develops *pari passu* a feeling of envy and of inferiority toward those among his own age-peers who continue the struggle and especially toward his own age-peers. Yet neither of these is the main source of the attacks. I have known many such dropouts, and I have even had the privilege of studying a small sample analytically. Not many are merely running from their critics, although the temptation to do so is strong. My impression is rather that most of those who run away from treating psychiatric patients are unwittingly running away from themselves, ie, from those aspects of themselves with which the psychotherapeutic entanglement confronts and challenges them. It is this selfconfrontation which disturbs the psychotherapist most deeply, whether young or old.

It is not strange then that in spite of the high incidence of suicide and mental illness among psychiatrists, in our training programs almost no attention is paid to the fact that the psychotherapeutic involvement imposes complex emotional stresses on all therapists, but especially on the younger men? Every patient who is undergoing psychotherapy of any kind requires high investments of feeling and time: *time* because change and growing up take time[3] and *feeling* because of the therapist's inescapable, mixed identifications with the patient, subtly masked though these may be. In varying degrees, therefore, each patient is a projection of the therapist's own buried self-images and of the unresolved conflicts associated with distortions of his self-image. In fact, each patient becomes a more or less symmetrical, mobile, animated, three-dimensional, unconscious Rorschach projection of the therapist, a composite of true perceptions and misperceptions with superimposed projections and identifications. As a result, and whether we realize this or not, when we treat someone else we are also treating or at least defending ourselves. This takes a great deal out of the therapist at any age, but especially when he is young.

In our present system of psychiatric training our residents are pitched headlong into this maelstrom while they are still emotionally immature and technically unschooled.[1,14] We force them to take this step before they have had adequate time or opportunity either for spontaneous emotional growth and change or for appropriate psychotherapeutic aids to growth. Is it strange then that this self-confrontation should stir tension and anxiety against which the student of psychiatry struggles to build up whatever defenses he can muster? (In analytic training, the "preparatory" or "training" analysis provides only a partial answer to this problem.)

In psychiatric residencies this struggle often produces brief but serious symptomatic episodes, which are rarely acknowledged and almost never discussed openly or searchingly. I have known seemingly solid young residents who reacted to their first experiences in psychotherapy by developing a wide variety of neurotic symptoms, eg, a true anorexia nervosa, compulsive eating, a mucous colitis, a painful, obstinate spastic colitis. I have known three who during their first weeks of service on a ward which was filled with actively disturbed psychotic patients wet and soiled their beds at night, for the first and only times since early childhood. Others developed potency disturbances. I recall two gifted residents who committed suicide, and others who committed suicide much later. Such upsets as these should arouse active concern in us as teachers because if a resident were to receive appropriate help *at that time* he would develop greater strength, empathy, and understanding out of his own painful reactions.

Under these circumstances is it not especially unfortunate that the accepted tradition among supervisors is to pride themselves on deliberately paying no attention to the therapeutic needs of their residents? As a result of this neglect almost no resident receives therapeutic help, even when he needs it as an integral part of his training.

Yet I am equally concerned about the resident who sails through his residency unshaken, seeming to feel nothing, usually imagining that to feel anything is *infra dig,* or that is will betray a "countertransference" which will get him into trouble.[15]

As long as teachers and supervising psychiatrists pretend that such problems do not exist or are not relevant, the resident will take his cues from the senior's attitude and will hide his symptoms and his suffering lest he lost his job and thus jeopardize his career. He will fear that frankness will delay his advancement. What the teacher blinds himself to and never mentions, the resident will be ashamed to acknowledge or discuss, thinking of his inner upset as unique. He concludes that whether they are natural or not, his own affective responses must be hidden. How then can the educators of these residents ever learn of the existence of such disturbances, much less help them? It seems obvious that no matter how burdensome and inconvenient this may be for us in our role as teachers, we must accept this therapeutic responsibility as educators.

Furthermore, the bland resident is the one who later on will hide behind curtains of cold, ironic indifference or sarcasm, the so-called *"banter" technique,* and, in the end, behind a depreciating attitude toward the task itself. Another will defend himself in an opposite way, ie, by burying his anger under excessive compassion. Either of these defenses may gain the approval of teachers, even as they stunt the resident's further growth. Sooner or later such a resident turns against psychiatry and psychotherapy. In many instances the effects remain dormant for years, only to appear later in hostility to patients, in rationalizations for overcharging them, in running away, and in suicides.

In recent years this early flight from the challenge of the patient has been encouraged in many ways by official psychiatric policies. If this continues, it will create a major obstacle to the development of new generations of mature psychiatrists in our time. (It may be illuminating to compare the situation in psychiatry with its counterpart in education. It is as difficult to measure results in education as in psychiatry, as difficult to characterize results qualitatively or even to determine *when* we should attempt an evaluation of results [ie, whether during the course of the educational process, or immediately after its formal termination, or five or ten or twenty years later]. These difficulties parallel closely the difficulties of evaluating psychiatric therapy. Yet there are also some interesting differences. Even among teachers who admit the existence of these difficulties, few use them as an excuse for withdrawing from the field of education. Even fewer use them as an excuse for maintaining that there is no such thing as education. And none uses them as an excuse for turning on education, educators, and students to attack them. Some may attack the tradition-bound thinking of other educators and the excessive claims or complacency of some but this does not constitute an attack on education itself. Yet this is what the dropout from psychotherapy is doing when he turns on psychotherapy, denies its very existence, and attacks it and those who practice it.[16])

Further Reasons for and Forms of Flight

As I said above, to treat patients intensively always stirs up pain, and pain always triggers an impulse to run away. This is not unlike the natural impulse to flee from battle and it is similarly condemned by our consciences, both conscious and unconscious. Usually this conflict is fought out in secret; and whether or not the individual runs away will depend upon the cumulative effects of many intrapsychic and psychosocial influences.

There are other and subtler intrapsychic reasons for this pain-driven flight from patients, about which I have written elsewhere.[14,16,17]

In addition to the activation of the therapist's own unsolved problems he faces a constant battering from the patient's overt or masked demands, or both, and often from the hostility of both the patient and the patient's family. In some measure they stir in the therapist his own incompletely resolved conflicts about his own family. The older man will have had enough years to acquire a lessened sensitivity to all of this and some devices for masking it. The younger man can protect himself only by withdrawing. His impulse to do this is natural. But where then does he turn? Inevitably he will turn to those forms of psychiatric activity which are relatively free from emotionally charged contacts with *individual* patients. Since there is some protection in numbers, even before he has learned how to deal with the problems of one patient he may turn to group therapy.[15,18] Or, he may turn to family therapy. Here, unfortunately, the family often takes a beating from the familial hostilities and sibling rivalries which the young psychiatrist does not recognize in himself and, therefore, visits on the patient's family. Or, he may turn to teaching: teaching *not* what he has learned out of his own struggles and out of his own experiences, but what as a medical student or young intern he had been told by others. Or there are those forms of research in which human involvement is at a minimum to which he can turn, especially where the research is at a minimum to which he can turn, especially where the research is on lower animals rather than on man. Another possibility open to him is the application of psychiatry to the community's needs, where he can indulge a hope that before he has mastered either himself or his techniques in dealing with one sick patient, he can "run a show" in a community mental health center for bringing healing to many. If he can recruit the personnel, he will administer an organization of nurses, psychologists, social workers, and still younger psychiatrists. He will make big plans, preside at conferences, and go on official trips.[17] These are attractive prospects. For meaningful but disturbing involvement with an individual he substitutes brief greetings as he passes down a line of waiting patients, a few quick words of interrogation, and then some words of "wisdom." These may be gratifying to his self-esteem, but at the same time he will be fending off that interaction with individual patients from which he should be learning to become a psychiatrist. Therefore, his growth stops here. The young man who retreats prematurely from work with individual patients, whether he retreats to work with groups or with families, or who turns prematurely to teaching, research, or the administration of community services, will never himself attain clinical maturity. All of these tasks have their intrinsic values. What they lack is intensive involvement with individuals, thus creating an anomalous culture of nongrowth by rewarding the student psychiatrist for turning his back on the essential challenge of the field which he professes to want to master. I repeat, therefore, that if we persist in seducing the young psychiatrist away from the individual patient into any of these adjuvant fields before he has matured in his ability to deal with interactions between his own emotional problems and those of individual patients, we will do his growth, his maturational processes, his empathy with illness, and, therefore, the whole future of psychiatry irreparable harm. (The issue here is not whether group and family therapies have values alone and as adjuvants to individual therapy. The evidence for this is convincing, provided only that it is not introduced so early in the sequence of training that it is vulnerable to misuse as an opportunity to run away. Actually the experience of many observers indicates[15] that some problems can be brought into clear perspective more rapidly in the privacy of individual psychotherapy but must later be resolved in group therapy[18]; whereas other problems can best be highlighted first in group or family therapy, but in the end must be fully worked out individually as well. Note that in both instances I do not say "always"; again because the approach to this question by both sides has been biased by too little tough-minded, hard-thinking skepticism. The question is not whether these approaches have value but how to avoid their misuse too early in any training program, so as not to turn them into opportunities to escape close involvement with individual patients. Many years ago I pointed to the lack of statistical studies to indicate how much economy of psychotherapeutic time or personnel is achieved in this way. One cannot deny the possibility that group processes may save some time and some personnel, but this hope still expresses more wishful thinking and optimism than factual data.)

There is still another particularly seductive form of flight from patients. This is the flight into a premature professorship. The promising young psychiatrist who is appointed to a professorship and to the chairmanship of his own department always starts out with a firm resolve never to stop treating a "few" patients. What actually happens, however, is so constant as to be predictable. First, the number of patients which constitute for him "the irreducible few" gradually dwindles. Then as more and more therapeutic appointments have to be cancelled by the psychiatrist because of the many other legitimate official demands on his time, his conscience begins to hurt. (The more conscientious he is, the more it hurts.) Finally, after passing through various phases, he throws in the sponge and quits all practice. One wrote me, "I have finally had to accept the fact that I have become one of the expendables." Another wrote, "Maybe I can dissuade other younger men from accepting these soul-destroying, careeristic promotions." (All of this brings to mind Alan Gregg's quotation from the younger Ostwald, who on a visit to this country commented that the Americans have a strange custom. They take a young man who has shown great promise in some field, and promote him to a higher position in which it is impossible for him to continue doing that in which he has shown such promise.[19])

Others are less honest and hide from their feelings of guilt behind a defensive barrier of scorn and sometimes of venom against any kind of psychotherapy.

This form of flight has serious consequences because younger men imitate their chiefs not only in flight, but also in pretending that flight is a gesture of moral superiority.

By its very nature especially in psychiatry the attainment of clinical maturity takes a long time, longer perhaps than any other form of training.[3, 20] Yet once a young man with relatively little clinical experience has accepted the chairmanship and professorship in any clinical department, he will find that his time is literally devoured by an increasing load of conflicting obligations. Furthermore, if his new post requires clinical maturity, no matter how great is his potential for growth as a clinician he will have little time to grow by working with patients in a consistent and sustained fashion, no time to lie fallow and ruminate about his experiences with patients, no time to change and grow with the changes and growth of patients. In spite even of a great potential for clinical growth, he will not, therefore, have time to grow up to his job. This is why no realist will say that a young departmental chief can learn to become a clinician *after* he has been appointed to such a job, whether this is in internal medicine, pediatrics, or psychiatry. He must have achieved his clinical maturity before accepting heavy administrative and pedagogic responsibilities. He will need this clinical maturity if he is ever to become a mature clinical professor and admin-

istrator, a director of the clinical work of others, or able
to inform clinical research with clinically mature judgment. The present tendency to appoint young men to
such posts before they have achieved clinical maturity is
a destructive trend. It will have to be reversed in psychiatry and indeed in all other clinical disciplines.

Where Then Can the Student of Psychiatry Become a Psychiatrist?

Maturing interactions with the struggles of individual
patients can be experienced in any setting which encourages prolonged, sustained, and intensive relationships
with a few patients at a time, for whose treatment one
carries full responsibility. (There is an additional virtue
in interspersing this with period of briefer surveys and
interactions, so that the student can make repeated
comparisons of both types of challenge.) In the past this
experience occurred primarily if not exclusively in
private practice. This is why under appropriate leadership private practice was for so many years our major
source of knowledge. Today this type of experience can
occur also on the inpatient and outpatient services of a
few psychiatric hospitals, but not in all; in some schools
and colleges, but not in all; in some units for industrial
psychiatry and in some social and penal agencies, but
not in all.

Each of these settings has its special advantages, but
also its disadvantages and limitations. For example,
private practice allows the therapist all the time he
needs. It also challenges him to carry his own load, to
accept personal responsibility, and to have the courage
and strength to make his own decisions without falling
back on the authority of a large prestigious institution.
The clinic and the hospital provide invaluable opportunities for concurrent observations by many simulta-
neous observers, which facilitate mutual scrutiny and
mutual comparison and criticism. None of this is readily
possible in the relative isolation of private practice.
Schools, industrial, penal, and social agencies provide opportunities to compare the influences of varied ethnic,

cultural, educational, and economic settings on the origins and incidence of the neurotic process, on its course, and on its responses to therapeutic maneuvers. These differences are obvious and well-known, but they are worth spelling out here if only to make it clear once more that each has its advantages and limitations. What I am stressing is that if it is to be possible to take full advantage of these settings, each must provide time enough for repeated, prolonged, sustained, and unhurried relationships between the man who is learning to become a psychiatrist and a few individual patients for whose intensive treatment he is responsible.

I know of only one setting in which it is literally impossible to become a psychiatrist, ie, in which neither clinical nor human maturation can occur. This is the setting which uses only an assembly-line approach to patients and where the official attitude is to scorn sustained individual interactions, and to take pride in brief interviews and a rapid turnover. Such institutions have no educational value. In fact, they mislead and misinform by perpetuating traditional clichés which are based on hasty impressions of brief cross-sections of a process which in reality must by its very nature be long drawn out.

If they are honest, the scientific leaders of such facilities acknowledge that a rapid turnover serves only to impress the more ignorant among legislators, and only those members of boards of trustees and those hospital and school administrators who are penny-wise and pound-foolish. It is a tragic error to rush patients in and out under the influence of the currently prevalent illusion that a quick turnover is economical and therefore desirable.

The effect on training of this rapid turnover is catastrophic; and young residents who have a sincere desire to learn soon leave such hospitals if they have the courage and the resources. Anyone who finds that he has stepped unwittingly into such a hospital starts at once to hunt around for some other residency where he can learn by working with patients at the slow pace which growth requires.[3, 20] Consequently the "quickie" hospitals end up staffed exclusively by medical hacks who do not care. I have seen such hospitals! Today, however, most young residents have families to support. Economic pressure makes it difficult for them to seek new jobs, however educationally advantageous these would be, especially since the hospitals with the poorer training frequently pay the higher salaries. (They have to, in order to recruit a staff.) Furthermore, even if a young resident has been tactful about his dissatisfaction with the policies of the hospital which he wants to leave, the administration will usually resent his leaving because it is so hard for them to find replacements. Consequently they often give the departing resident unfair, damaging references. I have seen and fought such so-called "references." They tend to keep many promising young men chained to destructive posts. I have known able young men who were trapped in this bind. The result is that before they have even had a chance to become psychiatrists they may be forced out of the field entirely.

This is a type of flight from patients which is imposed on residents against their will by defects in our training processes and by the selfishness, shortsightedness, and political expediency of some administrators.

REFERENCES

1. Kubie LS: Traditionalism in psychiatry. *J. Nerv Ment Dis* 139:6-19, 1964.

2. Kubie LS: The future of the private psychiatric hospital, in Gibson RW (ed): *Crosscurrents in Psychiatry and Psychoanalysis.* Philadelphia, JB Lippincott Co, 1967, pp. 179-203.

3. Kubie LS: The maturation of psychiatrists or the time that changes take. *J Nerv Ment Dis* 135:286-288, 1962.

4. Kubie LS: The neurotic potential, the neurotic process, and the neurotic state. *US Armed Forces Med J* 2:1-12, 1951.

5. Kubie LS: The distortion of the symbolic process in neurosis and psychosis. *J Amer Psychoanal Assoc* 1:59-86, 1953.

6. Kubie LS: The concept of normality and neurosis, in Heiman M (ed): *Psychoanalysis and Social Work,* New York, International Universities Press Inc, 1953, pp. 3-14.

7. Kubie LS: The fundamental nature of the distinction between normality and neurosis. *Psychoanal Quart* 23:167-204, 1954.

8. Kubie LS: The neurotic process as the focus of physiological and psychoanalytic research. *J Ment Sci* 104:519-536, 1958.

9. Kubie LS: Neurosis and normality, in Deutsch A (ed): *The Encyclopedia of Mental Health*. Philadelphia, F Franklin Watts Inc, 1963, vol 4, pp 1346-1353.

10. Kubie LS: The relation of psychotic disorganization to the neurotic process. *J Ameri Psychoanal Assoc* 15:626-640, 1967.

11. Kubie LS: Frontiers of research in psychiatry, in Redlich FC, Klerman GL, McDonald RK, et al (eds): *The University and Community Mental Health*. New Haven, Conn, Yale University Press, pp. 71-80.

12. Kubie LS: Missing and wanted: Heterodoxy in psychiatry and psychoanalysis. *J Nerv Ment Dis* 137:311, 1963.

13. Barzun J: *American University: How It Runs, Where It Is Going*. New York, Harper & Row Publishers Inc, 1968.

14. Kubie LS: Reflections on training, with discussions. *Psychoanal Forum* 1:95-112, 1966.

15. Kubie LS: The psychiatrist—his training and development. *Psychoanal Quart* 24:128-130, 1953.

16. Kubie LS: The psychotherapeutic ingredient in the learning process, in Porter R (ed): *The Role of Learning Psychotherapy*. London, J & A Churchill Ltd, 1968.

17. Kubie LS: Pitfalls of community psychiatry. *Arch Gen Psychiat* 18:257-266, 1968.

18. Kubie LS: Some theoretical concepts underlying the relationship between individual and group psychotherapies. *Int J Group Psychother* 8:3-19, 1958.

19. Gregg A: *The Furtherance of Medical Research* (The Terry Lectures). New Haven, Conn, Yale University Press, 1941.

20. Kubie LS: The problem of maturity in psychiatric research. *J Med Educ* 28:11-27, 1953.

NEW APPROACHES
TO MENTAL ILLNESS:
THE FAILURE
OF A TRADITION

H. J. Eysenck

It is probably true to say that until quite recently American Psychiatry, particularly in so far as it was concerned with neurotic disorders, presented a fairly monolithic approach; clinical psychology followed suit, and certainly did not present any particular challenge to this program. Basic to the psychiatric approach was some form of psychoanalytic theory, attributing neurotic disorders to early childhood events, repression, the growth of complexes, and the emergence of symptoms which were relatively unimportant and merely indicated the existence of serious underlying difficulties. In line with this theory, treatment was by preference psychoanalytic, i.e., long-term, interpretive interaction between therapist and patient; when not classically psychoanalytic, treatment was nevertheless predicated on the truth of the psychoanalytic theory, and imitated the main features of such treatment as far as possible. Nurses, social workers, and clinical treatment as far as possible. Nurses, social workers, and clinical psychologists—indeed, everybody who was connected with the psychiatric team in any way, shape, or form was indoctrinated with psychoanalytic beliefs and played his or her part in the joint endeavor. There were, of course, many departures from analytic orthodoxy, but on the whole the underlying ideas did not change too drastically. In so far as psychology made any contribution, it was by stressing the importance of projective

95

devices, such as the Rorschach and T.A.T. tests; the major use of these was to help in the elucidation of psychoanalytic mechanisms. Diagnosis and biological factors were decried, and environmental factors, particularly of a familial kind, were stressed almost exclusively. Withall, great claims were made for the success of this system, and all alternative methods were declared worthless; at best, they might provide temporary therapy for symptoms, but even then the patient would be faced with relapse or symptom substitution. His general outlook, therefore, was gloomy; without therapy, he would never recover; to obtain proper (analytic) therapy, he had to give up much time and a great deal of money—without any guarantee of success even then.

These claims and beliefs were almost universally accepted, and the whole system of training of psychiatrists in the U. S. A. was based on the correctness of this view. Yet it would seem that in every particular this system of beliefs and hypotheses is in fact wrong. Neurotics tend in the majority of cases to improve dramatically without any therapeutic intervention by psychiatrists or psychologists (spontaneous remission); when treated by psychoanalysis or some similar form of psychotherapy, patients do not improve more quickly than when not treated psychiatrically at all; when symptoms are removed by some form of treatment alternative to analysis (such as behavior therapy) there are neither relapses nor symptom substitutions. No lengthy treatment is in fact required; modern methods of behavior therapy effect cures in severe cases of complex neurotic illness in an average of 30 sessions, and often phobic and other types of neurotic illness are cleared up in five sessions, or even less. Projective tests have been found to be unreliable and invalid; instead, tests of biological functioning (autonomic reactivity, eyeblink conditioning, G. S. R. habituation, etc.) have been found increasingly useful; Martin et al. (1969) have shown, for instance, that the relative success of psychotherapy and of behavior therapy can be predicted with considerable success from knowledge of the patient's speed of eyeblink conditioning. A brief review of the literature may be useful in substantiating some of these claims.

In 1952, the writer published a paper in which he examined closely the evidence which had been published up to that date regarding the claims for psychotherapeutic effectiveness of analytic and other methods. He pointed out that what was required, first of all, was a base-line against which to measure such effectiveness, i.e., some estimate of how well severely ill neurotics would progress without any psychiatric help at all. Reviewing the evidence available at the time, he came to the conclusion that spontaneous remission was an undoubted fact; marked remission or complete cure was claimed for untreated neurotics with severe symptoms in some 70% after 2 years, and in some 90% in all after 5 years without treatment other than ordinary, nonpsychiatric G. P. treatment. Much further work has been published on this point since then, and has been reviewed repeatedly (Eysenck, 1960, 1969); the latest review has been published in book form by S. Rachman (1971). This book provides a very detailed examination of all the available studies, critically examining the strength and weakness of each, and judiciously combining the most important and relevant ones to give us the most acceptable conclusion as of now. It may be worthwhile to quote his conclusion:

> "the available evidence does not permit a revision of Eysenck's (1952) estimate of a gross spontaneous remission rate of approximately 65% of neurotic disorders over a two-year period. However, the evidence which has been presented since the original estimate was attempted, emphasizes the need for more refined studies and more accurate statistics. In particular, it is now possible to say with a high degree of certainty that the gross spontaneous remission rate is not constant across different *types* of neurotic disorder. It is for example, probable that obsessional disorders show a lower rate of spontaneous remission than anxiety conditions. Future investigators would be well advised to analyse the spontaneous remission rates of the various neuroses within rather than across diagnostic groupings. If we proceed in this manner it should eventually be possible to make more accurate estimates of the likelihood of spontaneous remission occurring in a particular type of disorder and indeed for a particular group of patients.

Although the gross spontaneous remission rate has thus far been based on a two-year period of observation (and this serves well for many purposes), attempts to understand the nature of the process will, of course, be facilitated by an extension of the periods of observation. The collection of reliable observations on the course of spontaneous remission will, among other things, greatly assist in making prognoses.

Naturally, the determination of a reliable rate of spontaneous remission is only the first stage in a process of exploration. Both for its own sake and for practical reasons, we need to approach an understanding of the causes of spontaneous remission. Eysenck (1963) has adumbrated a theory to account for remissions and relapses which draws attention to the possible role of individual differences in personality. In addition, there are numerous bits of incidental information pertinent to the subject which are contained in clinical reports, follow-up studies and the like (e.g. Stevenson, 1961). Respondents who have recovered from neurotic disorders often attribute their improvements to the occurrence of fortunate *events*. Some of the more commonly mentioned are financial gains, improvements in occupation, successful marriages and personal relationships, the amelioration of pressing difficulties, and so on (e.g. Friess and Nelson, 1942; Imber *et al.*, 1968). The identification of these restorative events and study of the manner in which they affect the process of remission would be of considerable value.

Unfortunately the encouragement which can be derived from the occurrence of spontaneous remissions in neuroses must be tempered by recognition of the fact that a sizeable minority of patients do not remit spontaneously. Approximately one third of all neurotic patients do not improve spontaneously and it could be that in future, it is this group of people who will absorb the attentions of clinicians and research workers. Such a redirection of effort must, of course, depend upon an accurate system of identification and prognosis. The size of the problem can be estimated from the current rates of rejection, defection and failure reported by psychotherapists."

Eysenck (1952) went on to compare the claimed effectiveness of psychotherapy with the base-line so established. Such a comparison is, of course, beset with many difficulties. Patients treated with psychoanalysis are very highly selected on the basis of education, youth, income, and generally favorable prognosis; on these grounds alone they should do better than the "spontaneous remission" sample. Again, the only judges of the success or failure of the patients treated by psychoanalysis and psychotherapy generally were the therapists themselves, and there is evidence to suggest that these may have been prejudiced in favor of their own success. Last, there is the well-known "hello—good-bye" effect; patients may enter therapy on the down-swing of their periodic illness attacks, and leave on the up-swing, with the therapist claiming the difference as due to his own efforts, rather than a natural change in status; only long-term follow-up procedures, conspicuously missing from the data, could sort out this type of effect. There are other difficulties; no control groups (untreated or treated by other methods) were provided by the psychotherapists who published their own figures, and it is difficult if not impossible to compare standards of "improvement" or "cure," or of initial "illness," from one study to another. Having drawn attention to these and other problems, Eysenck (1952) completed his calculations and showed that the figures for improvement and cure claimed by psychotherapists were almost identical with those found for the untreated cases; about 2 out of 3 recovered after treatment probably lasting on the average about 2 years! In other words, there was in all this no evidence at all of therapeutic success over and above the spontaneous remission rate. It would have been wrong to claim that these figures proved psychotherapy to be ineffective, and no such claim was made; it was concluded that the figures failed to support any claim for therapeutic usefulness of psychotherapy. (Many critics have disregarded the careful wording of the article, and have accused the writer of making the unjustified claim that psychotherapy had in fact been proved to be useless. The outcome of the comparison was sufficiently dramatic to make far-reaching and exaggerated claims of this kind quite unnecessary, and none were in fact made.) Again, many studies have been reported in the years which have elapsed since this early paper was published (Eysenck, 1960, 1969), but they have only served to reinforce the conclusions drawn then; even now, there is in existence no study which clearly and without reasonable doubt gives evidence of therapeutic superiority of psychoanalysis or psychotherapy over no treatment, or alternative treatment such as behavior therapy, in comparably chosen groups of patients. Rachman (1971) sums up his careful and balanced survey by saying: "It is disappointing to find that the best studies of psychotherapy yield discouraging results while the inadequate studies are over-optimistic. . . . There is still no acceptable evidence to support the view that psychoanalytic treatment is effective."

What about the possibility that psychotherapy may actually do harm to patients? This question has been raised by a number of persons working within the Rogerian framework, notably Truax and Carkhuff (1967); they argue that the over-all failure of psychotherapy to do better than spontaneous remission is not due to its absolute lack of power, but rather that, depending on his personality, the psychotherapist may make the patient better, or he may make the patient worse—the two cancelling out when you consider the average effect. The requisite personality characteristics for successful therapy are warmth, empathy, and genuineness; given these, any system of psychotherapy is declared to work. Without them, any system will make the patient worse. Rogerians have declared these three conditions of effective psychotherapy to be "necessary and sufficient," but in recent years further conditions have been suggested, such as "self-exploration" and "persuasive potency." Rachman has surveyed the evidence critically, and has come to the conclusion that while interesting and suggestive, it is far from conclusive. He further suggests that in so far as there are elements of truth in it, the Rogerian approach to this problem could find an explanation in terms of behavior theory. He concludes his chapter in this way:

> "It is suggested that this type of approach could be facilitated by recasting the Rogerian approach in terms of learning theory. Truax and Carkhuff have in fact made the initial steps in this direction by proposing that therapists who are high on the three conditions are potent positive reinforcers. Similarly those therapists who are low on these qualities are ineffective or even negative reinforcers. They suggest that the potent therapist provides positive reinforcement of "approach responses to human relating," reinforcement of self-exploratory behaviour, the elim-

ination of specific fear, the "reinforcement of positive self-concepts and self-evaluations" (p. 151-152). Parts of this model bear some resemblance to Wolpe's (1958) view of non-systematic desensitization which he argues can be used to explain the fact that most forms of therapy are capable of producing at least some therapeutic successes. Similarly, the Truax and Carkhuff model is congruent with some of the views put forward by Krasner (1962) on the reinforcing powers of a therapist.

If the Rogerian research proceeds from this model, it should be possible to bring about a fruitful integration with behavioural techniques and the ensuing combination might be valuable."

We have so far only considered therapy with neurotic adults; similar results are found when we consider therapy with children, and therapy with psychotic adults (Rachman, 1971). The evidence throughout fails to give any support whatever to psychoanalytic claims for therapeutic effectiveness; indeed, psychotherapy of any kind fares badly when the results are compared with spontaneous remission. There are now a great number of studies available, many with control groups which make comparisons less hazardous than in the earlier days when diverse types of patients had to be compared since control groups proper were lacking; yet the answer to our question has not changed one bit. Evidence for psycho-therapeutic effectiveness is still elusive, and the null hypothesis can still be maintained without any great difficulty. Gradually the truth of this generalization is being appreciated even by doctrinaire psychotherapists who keep in touch with literature, and claims are being scaled down to read: "We don't claim to cure the patient; we enable him to live better with his symptoms, and/or we make him a better (more insightful) person." Such claims are meaningful only if they refer to measurable qualities (and no efforts have been made to measure the qualities here alluded to), and if there is no way of actually curing the patient of his symptoms. It is the writer's opinion that new methods are now available which do the trick, usually in a tenth or less of the time required by psychoanalysis to fail in doing it. These methods I have labelled "behavior therapy" (Eysenck, 1959); they are derived from modern learning theory, and contrast in many ways with those of psychotherapy. In particular, they are based on a different theory of neurosis than the Freudian; according to this view, there are no "complexes" underlying "symptoms" that require "interpretation" and "insight." Neurotic manifestations, erroneously called "symptoms," are simply conditioned emotional reactions and their somatic correlates and effects; a cure consists in the extinction of these conditioned responses (Eysenck, 1960, 1964). Table 1 sets out in some detail the main differences between these two views.

To many people the derivation of the methods of behavior therapy from modern learning theory and the large amount of laboratory work with humans and animals supporting its various generalizations are of little concern. These people are more interested in the simple question: does behavior therapy produce more and quicker cures than psychotherapy?

In this form the question is probably unanswerable. We must specify the type of patient treated, his symptoms, and the length and severity of his disorder; we must specify the precise nature and dimensions of what is to be considered "cure"; we must specify the precise nature of methods to be used under the headings of "behavior therapy" and "psychotherapy," and the amount of training and expertise required of the therapists. Finally, we should ideally have several therapists on each side, so that we can evaluate the therapist's contribution to the variance as well as the method's contribution. Only limited steps have been taken to answer some of the questions included in this list. I will try to give some preliminary, tentative answers, based on the literature of the last ten years.

In summarizing relevant studies we must consider two ways of looking at the problem. The academic research worker is interested in the extension of certain general laws about conditioning and the extinction of habits, from their origin in the laboratory, to the clinic and the prison. The therapist is interested in the well-being and improvement of his patient. This difference affects many aspects of the problem; the type and rigor of the proof

TABLE 1

Psychotherapy	Behavior Therapy
1. Based on inconsistent theory never properly formulated in postulate form.	Based on consistent, properly formulated theory leading to testable deductions.
2. Derived from clinical observations made without necessary control observations or experiments.	Derived from experimental studies designed to test basic theory and deductions made therefrom.
3. Considers symptoms the visible up-shot of unconscious causes ("complexes").	Considers symptoms as unadaptive conditioned responses.
4. Regards symptoms as evidence of *repression.*	Regards symptoms as evidence of faulty learning.
5. Believes that symptomatology is determined by defense mechanisms.	Believes that symptomatology is determined by individual differences in conditionability and autonomic lability, as well as accidental environmental circumstances.
6. All treatment of neurotic disorders must be *historically* based.	All treatment of neurotic disorders is concerned with habits existing at *present;* their historical development is largely irrelevant.
7. Cures are achieved by the underlying (unconscious) dynamics, not by treating symptom itself.	Cures are achieved by treating the symptom itself, i.e., by extinguishing unadaptive C.Rs. and establishing desirable C.Rs.
8. Interpretation of symptoms, dreams, acts, etc., is an important element of treatment.	Interpretation, even if not completely subjective and erroneous, is irrelevant.
9. Symptomatic treatment leads to the elaboration of new symptoms.	Symptomatic treatment leads to permanent recovery provided autonomic as well as skeletal surplus C.Rs. are extinguished.
10. Transference relations are essential for cures of neurotic disorders.	Personal relations are not essential for cures of neurotic disorder, although they may be useful in certain circumstances.

demanded, the type of experimental subject or patient studied, and the nature of the measure of change in behavior used by the investigator. Recognition of this dif-

ference in approach is important because many incon-
clusive and irrelevant arguments have arisen from it,
arguments which simply illustrate that research psychologists and clinical psychiatrists do not necesarily
share the same aims and concerns.

Certain neurotic symptoms can be observed in otherwise fairly normal persons; indeed, normality and
neurosis constitute a continuum. Some of these symptoms, for example simple phobias, provide an exception-
ally clear-cut means of measuring the effects of treatment. Fears of snakes, spiders, public speaking, test-
taking, open or closed spaces, or heights, can be
measured with great precision, by actually placing the
subject in a situation in which he is required to go near a
snake, or go up a ladder; his behavior can be accurately
observed and measured, and can be shown to be very reliable and stable over time. Physiological measures of
fear can be taken, and correlated with behavior and self-
ratings of fear. This makes possible accurate measurement of pre- and post-therapy behavior, and allows us to
measure the effects of therapy, and to compare different
therapies. A dozen *laboratory research projects* since
1961 have used this method and about half of these have
also provided a follow-up period averaging eight to nine
months.

The type of behavior therapy used in all cases was Jo-
seph Wolpe's method of desensitization—the gradual introduction of the feared object while the patient is in a
state of relaxation; the feared object is introduced in
"hierarchies," first in a form that is not much feared,
later in a more direct or severe form. Control groups were
tested after no treatment, simple relaxation, flooding or
"implosion" of the feared object, suggestion and hypnosis, drug-placebo, or insight therapy; in all cases the
groups treated with behavior therapy showed greater
change in behavior, in the direction of lessening of fear,
than did the control groups.

Another advantage of this procedure is that it permits
us to study which aspects of the method used are most
important. Dr. Stanley Rachman's 1965 studies of relaxation without gradual use of hierarchies, hierarchies

without relaxation, and combined hierarchies and relaxation may be quoted here. He found that combined relaxation and hierarchies gave the best results. P. J.
Lang's 1969 studies on personal administration of desensitization therapy as compared with computer-adminis-
tered desensitization therapy are also relevant; he found
no difference. We may conclude from all these studies
that desensitization unquestionably has the effect of
lessening phobic fears of certain objects and situations
to a strikingly greater extent than other procedures used;
that both parts of the procedure (relaxation and hierarchies) seem necessary, and that impersonal methods
(computer) work as well as personal methods, contrary to
the hypothesis that "transference" effects are important.

Psychiatrists often object to experiments such as these
that monosymptomatic phobias are rare: that the subjects of these experiments are not neurotics of the kind
referred to clinics; and that the relevance of these demonstrations to their day-to-day work is doubtful. Such
relevance must of course be demonstrated, but it should
be added that for Freud and his followers even mild errors in performance and minor misspellings were
evidence of deep-seated complexes, and snake phobias in
particular were explained along symbolic lines which
linked them securely with his theoretical system; indeed,
it was for this reason that Lang and his associates selected snake phobics for their experiments. Psycho-
analysts cannot therefore have it both ways; either these
phobias are typical of more severe neurotic disorders, in
which case we may generalize from these results with
some confidence, or their original views were mistaken.
There is no doubt that Freud would not have predicted
that the methods used by behavior therapists would succeed in effectively curing these disorders, minor though
they might be; according to his set of hypotheses no
permanent eradication of such fears (without relapse or
symptom substitution) should be possible without "insight." The fact that results conclusively disprove this
Freudian notion should not be allowed to go by default; it
strongly argues against the whole psychoanalytic
theory.

The fact that in these experimental studies mono-symptomatic phobic patients have been used has given rise to the erroneous supposition (sometimes voiced as a criticism of behavior therapy) that these methods can deal *only* with monosymptomatic phobias. This is not true, as we shall see; the reason for concentrating on this type of patient is simply experimental convenience, and the possibility of accurate measurement of initial and final state. Mendel concentrated on wrinkled and smooth peas; but it does not follow that the laws of genetics he discovered only apply to wrinkled and smooth peas! Psychiatrists often fail to appreciate the value of having a convenient "test bed" for investigation rigorously and quantitatively the deductions from one's theories; be-havior therapy has for the first time made this approach feasible in the field of psychotherapy. This insistence on taking previously inaccessible problems into the labora-tory is perhaps the major contribution of behavior therapy to psychiatry.

Proof of the effectiveness of behavior therapy *using patients as subjects* in controlled comparisons is of course much less easy to give, particularly since psycho-analysts have been remarkably coy in refusing to take part in joint experimental studies comparing the effects of different types of therapy. However, a number of such studies have now been carried out, all of them from the Institute of Psychiatry at the Maudsley Hospital, and we can at least have a preliminary glimpse of the likely results of such comparisons.

The work done by John Cooper et al. (1965), Isaac Marks and Michael Gelder (1965), Gelder et al. (1967) and Marks et al. (1968) covers over 110 patients treated with desensitization-type behavior therapy, included follow-ups of about twelve months in every case, and used various "controls" (groups with similar conditions but differently treated, for subsequent comparison) ranging from simple hospitalization to mixed treatment, hypnotic suggestion, and insight psychotherapy. Some of these were retrospective studies, in which matching was at-tempted from case records; these showed that isolated phobias responded significantly better to desensitization than to control treatment; complex phobic disorders such as agoraphobia (fear of open spaces) did rather better, but not significantly so. Obsessive neuroses and a group of other miscellaneous neuroses did no better (but also no worse) with desensitization than with control treatment. In looking at these results it should be borne in mind that the behavior therapy in question was done by psychologists experimenting with new methods of their own devising. (In recent, unpublished work we have been able to show that for both these groups—agoraphobics and obsessionals—a different type of behavior therapy—"flooding" or implosion therapy—is both a quick and efficient method of treatment; gradually an understanding along theoretical lines is being developed as to when desensitization and when "flooding" is the appropriate method of treatment.)

Furthermore, patients selected for behavior therapy were usually only referred as a last resort, after all other methods had conspicuously failed; it is impossible to match for this feature. The fact that in spite of all these difficulties behavior therapy emerged as significantly superior in most cases, and inferior in none, must count as a startling success.

Studies designed to provide a control group demonstrated again the significant superiority of behavior therapy in out-patients with focal phobias or agoraphobia. Not only did the phobias improve, but, Marks and Gelder report, "once the treated phobias diminished improvements also followed in work and leisure adjustments that had formerly been hampered by the phobias." With a group of severely agoraphobic inpatients desensitization failed to do better than the control condition, but again it did no worse. The value of desensitization was found to be inversely proportional to the amount of severe free-floating anxiety in these cases; the more anxiety, the less successful the treatment, as compared to the control treatment.

Two recent and as yet unpublished studies have been carried out by Ph.D. students in my department, working under the direction of Dr. Stanley Rachman. In the first of these, Jim Humphrey allocated on a random basis successive child guidance cases suffering from neurotic disorders to treatment by either behavior therapy or psychotherapy; a nontreated control group was also available. Improvement was judged by two independent psychiatrists, ignorant of the treatment received: a ten month follow-up was also provided. Behavior therapy took much less time—18 weeks as compared with 31 weeks for psychotherapy, on average. Success of behavior therapy in improving the psychiatric condition of the child was significantly greater, in spite of the shorter time required. Unfortunately the children in the behavior therapy group, although matched by random procedures, were more seriously ill than the children in the psychotherapy group, this statistically significant difference partly invalidates the comparisons.

A similar, but rather more extensive study was done on adult patients by Patricia Gillan. Her patients were all out-patients suffering from serious and complex phobic anxieties; there were no monosymptomatic cases among her patients, many of whom in fact had difficulties in coming up to the hospital for treatment. She formed four groups of eight patients each, on a part random, part matching basis. Those in group 1 were given desensitization treatment with relaxation; those in group 2 were given the hierarchies, but no relaxation; those in group 3 were given relaxation, plus pseudo-therapy, but no hierarchies; those in group 4 were given dynamic psychotherapy by a psychiatrist. Patients were rated by the therapist involved, and also by an independent psychiatrist uncommitted to either approach, who formed his judgment "blind," i.e., in ignorance of which treatment had been administered. Physiological measures were taken of the amount of fear produced by the phobic object or situation, both at the end of therapy and after a follow-up period of three months.

The results of this work clearly favor behavior therapy. The combination of relaxation and hierarchies is the most successful form of treatment, with hierarchies without relaxation somewhat inferior, but not significantly so; psychotherapy and relaxation without hierarchies are both significantly inferior. These two studies of random samples of neurotic children and of adults with serious disorders suggest that the work reported from laboratory experiments can be replicated with psychiatric patients, and that we are justified in extending our conclusions from the one field to the other. This is an important advance.

The relatively high success of the method of using hierarchies, even without relaxation, fits well with another hypothesis I have put forward, namely that when psychotherapy is effective (though less so than behavior therapy) it is so because it incorporates certain principles of desensitization. The permissive atmosphere produces a lowering of anxiety (relaxation); discussion ranges around the presenting problems, and in the hands of an experienced psychiatrist naturally centers on problems towards the lower end of the hierarchy because these arouse only anxieties which under the circumstances are tolerable, to be followed later by discussions involving problems higher up the hierarchy.

Thus psychotherapy may often approach, though rather inefficiently because unintentionally, the procedure of hierarchy construction and working through, and thus resemble Gillan's second method (giving the hierarchies but no relaxation). Support for this notion comes from the clear demonstration of C. B. Truax and R. R. Carkhuff, already mentioned, that while some psychotherapists can be shown consistently to help their patients, others equally consistently not only fail to help but actively retard recovery; what is of interest here is their description of the personality qualities and "therapy styles" of these two contrasted groups of therapists. They find empathy, warmth, and genuineness characteristic of successful therapists (operational definitions of these terms are of course given); absence of these qualities, and in particular the presence of the opposites, is found in therapists who actually hurt and harm their patients. This is very much in line with my view of successful psychotherapy as embodying behaviorist principles; empathy, warmth, and genuineness generate an easy, relaxed atmosphere in which to develop the hierarchies which carry so much of the burden of successful therapy, while cold, "interpretive," and purist behavior on the part of the thrapist has the opposite effect, i.e., preventing relaxation and increasing anxiety. According to this theory, then, relaxation is usually present in interviews with "good" therapists and does not have to be created artificially by training, although such training may be necessary with some patients.

It may be worthwhile to pursue this theory a little further. The hypothetical process of "deconditioning" or extinction of habits involved in behavior therapy implies the formation of new conditioned responses, whether in behavior therapy or in psychotherapy; one might predict that subjects who form conditioned responses easily and quickly would do better in therapy than those who do so poorly and slowly. Irene Martin et al. (1969) have recently shown that those who quickly acquire eye-blink conditioned responses in the lab are much more likely to do well with both behavior therapy and psychotherapy; this strongly supports my view, as well as suggesting more widespread use of this test as a prognostic device. Certainly no projective or other widely used test has to my knowledge ever succeeded as well as this in predicting success of therapy.

The desensitization methods of behavior therapy are designed for neurotic, not psychotic disorders and I have put forward the view that psychoticism is a personality variable which works against therapeutic success, whether in psychotherapy or in behavior therapy; with people high on P, either drug therapy or behavior therapy through operant conditioning is required. The failure in the Marks and Gelder studies where in-patients are concerned may thus be due to the unsuspected presence of a P component; certainly this failure was as marked in psychotherapy as in behavior therapy.

I have concentrated on desensitization methods, for the simple reason that trials using control groups are almost nonexistent outside this field. There are isolated exceptions, such as the 1969 paper by I. G. Thompson and N. H. Rathod dealing with aversion therapy in heroin addiction; using scoline injection which produces muscular paralysis and fear of suffocation as the unconditioned response, they elaborated a conditioning procedure in which self-injection with heroin just prior to paralysis constituted the conditioned stimulus. This method worked very well, as compared with a not too satisfactory control group. The severity of the effect of using scoline is justified by the poor prognosis of heroin addicts—after five years, untreated addicts are likely to be dead. The study needs replication, of course, but in view of the well-known lack of effect of other types of treatment the results must be considered as extremely promising—eight out of ten patients did not use heroin after treatment, as checked by frequent urine analyses carried out without prior warning.

In their book *Aversion Therapy and Behavior Disorders,* Stanley Rachman and John Teasdale make the point that in most disorders where aversion therapy is attempted (alcoholism, homosexuality, fetishism, transvestism, drug addiction) the spontaneous remission rate and the success rate of other methods of treatment are reasonably well known, and are both so low that any sizeable number of "cures," even though they may need booster doses of treatment, may be regarded as highly suggestive, although proper proof with use of control groups must of course remain the ideal. They demonstrate that aversion therapy can be made to work extremely well *provided* that the laws of established laboratory procedures for conditioning and habit extinction are not flouted in the process—as is too often done by psychiatrists not too knowledgeable in this field, and eager to apply methods whose rationale they comprehend only imperfectly.

Some studies have shown that expectation of improvement (Harold Leitenberg et al., 1969) or knowledge of the therapeutic intention of the procedure (S. Miller, unpublished) may be essential to success. The former study showed that the effects of desensitization were significantly impaired when expectation of improvement was removed; in the latter, subjects working under the impression that they were participating in an experiment on "imagery" showed significantly less effect than others who knew that the object of the experiment was therapeutic. This knowledge had to be present from the beginning; when it was imparted just before testing for the effects of treatment, effects were minimal. These experiemts suggest the presence of reinforcement in desensitization, possibly mediated by the therapist's praise and approval (real or imagined), or by "knowledge of results." These effects might repay closer study.

A summing-up at present must be tentative. It is important to note that in all the 20 or so studies using control groups, whether dealing with experimental analogue "patients" or with real psychiatric cases, behavior therapy did significantly better than psychotherapy, or any other alternative method, in almost every case; it never did worse. When you remember that the behavior therapists in question were usually psychologists with little training in the method, and little experience (often Ph.D. students who had just a few hours of instruction), or else people experimenting with new and not yet worked-out methods, then you may begin to feel, as I do, that this result is really astonishingly positive and almost incredible; there is nothing like it in the history of psychiatry. It is possible to find fault with details of individual studies, and to suspend judgment in the case of others; it is very difficult to look at the evidence as a whole (which is of course what a scientist should do!) and come to any other conclusion than that behavior therapy not only has been shown to work, but that it is the *only* method of psychological therapy for which this can be claimed. This seems to me the one conclusion which has been very firmly established; we do not as yet know which types of patients it works best for (although some indications for this have been mentioned), we do not know which of several theories regarding the method of working of desensitization is correct (although some evidence is beginning to come in), and we do not know how to predict success or failure (although the work on eye-blink conditioning has laid a firm basis for research in this field). These may seem a large number of "don't knows," but in view of the youth of the methods of behavior therapy we may perhaps rather congratulate ourselves on the fact that its clinical and scientific value and usefulness have been so firmly established.

Desensitization, aversion therapy, and "flooding" are only three of the many techniques which have been elaborated by behavior therapists; another one is "modeling" (Bandura, 1969), which has many claims to our attention. It is the only technique which has ever, in a properly controlled trial, proved superior to desensitization, and it has a good background in experimental psychology. There is no doubt that in the next few years much more will be heard of this technique.

For psychotics, operant techniques deriving from Skinner have proved of greater use than the methods which have been shown to have therapeutic value in neurotics. Ullman and Krasner (1969) give a good summary of much of the work done with schizophrenics and autistic children, in particular. In addition to individual studies, there has also been a major breakthrough in the group treatment of deteriorated schizophrenics; the "token economy" (Ayllon and Azrin, 1968) has been used with great effectiveness in retraining patients long since given up by psychiatrists, and produces reversions to normality of astonishing size. This is not the place to discuss any of these techniques or effects in detail; the references cited will help the reader to look up areas in which he is particularly interested.

To complete our account of the failure of the old tradition, let me just mention in passing that the major diagnostic and pretherapeutic tool of old-fashioned psychiatry, the projective test, has also been found wanting, and is being replaced by more appropriate techniques. Here is a summary of a review of results achieved with projective devices (Eysenck, 1958); none of these results would seem to require change in view of the more recent, and very thorough, review given by Zubin, Eron, and Schumer, 1965.

"(i) There is no consistent, meaningful and testable theory underlying modern projective devices. (ii) The actual practice of projective experts frequently contradicts the putative hypotheses on which their tests are built. (iii) On the empirical level, there is no indisputable evidence showing any kind of marked relationship between global projective test interpretation by experts, and psychiatric diagnosis. (iv) There is no evidence of any marked relationship between Rorschach scoring categories combined in any approved statistical fashion into a scale, and diagnostic category, when the association between the two is tested on a population other than that from which the scale was derived. (v) There is no evidence of any marked relationship between global or statistically derived projective test scores, and outcome of psychotherapy. (vi) There is no evidence for the great majority of the postulated relationships between projective test indicators and personality traits. (vii) There is no evidence for any marked relationship between projective test indicators of any kind and intellectual qualities and abilities as measured, estimated, or rated independently. (viii) There is no evidence for the predictive power of projective techniques with respect to success or failure in a wide variety of fields where personality qualities play an important part. (ix) There is no evidence that conscious or unconscious conflicts, attitudes, fears, or fantasies in patients can be diagnosed by means of projective techniques in such a way as to give congruent results with assessments made by psychiatrists independently. (x) There is ample evidence to show that the great majority of studies in the field of projective techniques are inadequately designed, have serious statistical errors in the analysis of the data, and/or are subject to damaging criticisms on the grounds of contamination between test and criterion."

What is the alternative, as far as diagnostic and predictive personality testing is concerned? If we regard the patient, for therapeutic purposes, as a biological mechanism which has temporarily gone wrong and requires either the extinction of acquired emotional responses, or else the acquisition of new, more appropriate ones (Eysenck, 1967), then clearly tests of conditioning (the ease of forming conditioned responses, their strength, their rate of extinction), habituation, autonomic responsiveness, etc. are needed, and we have already mentioned that simple eye-blink conditioning measures predict with considerable accuracy the effectiveness of desensitization and psychotherapy (Martin et al., 1969). Furthermore, these various methods of measuring autonomic responsiveness to specific stimuli give us a much-needed chance of following in considerable detail the progress of therapy, and of checking on the theory, according to which certain consequences of treatment can be predicted (see the papers of Marks and Gelder, for example). In this way a rational link can be built up between diagnosis, therapy, and effectiveness of treatment; such links help us greatly in coming to rational decisions about the value of a given therapy, and of a given theory. Consider for example the very specific way in which we can decondition the separate parts of a given transvestite fetishist's perversions; aversion therapy involving panties removes this particular article of clothing from his list (as checked by penis plethysmography), leaving other articles of clothing unimpaired. These can then be removed from his list one by one, always checking on the physiological effects of the treatment and demonstrating the success of the method for one item before going on to the next. It is these very specific proofs which render the theory so impressive.

There have of course been many criticisms of behavior therapy; I have discussed these at some length elsewhere (Eysenck, 1970). Arguments about relapses and symptom substitution, which were frequent in the early years, have now practically disappeared; too many patients have been treated and followed up without any trace of either of these consequences being found to make this a profitable point of discussion. Most arguments center on the point that what is done is merely "symptom removal"; but of course that is the central point of behavior therapy. According to our theory, the "symptom" *is* the "illness"; once it is removed there is nothing left! However that may be, it ill becomes those who cannot *even* remove the "symptom" to complain that behavior therapists cannot remove anything *but* the symptom!

It should be realized that behavior therapy is not an *addition* to orthodox psychotherapy; it is an *alternative*. Its advent has already produced a revolution in methods of treatment, and this revolution will soon substitute the new methods for the old, as more and more psychiatrists and clinical psychologists realize through observation and experience the powers of the new methods. Psychoanalysis has held psychiatry in thrall for over fifty years, preventing any new developments; this premature crystallization of spurious orthodoxy has had a most deleterious effect on treatment. Behavior therapy, even if its methods should turn out to be little better than those it seems destined to replace, has had the all-important effect of introducing a new, questioning attitude into this field; its insistence that all claims for therapeutic usefulness should be empirically demonstrated to be justified must have a beneficial effect where previously all was speculation and *ex cathedra* pronouncements.

Who is to do behavior therapy? Clearly these methods demand a background, and competence, in learning theory, conditioning methodology, social psychology, and other specialties which at the moment are not taught in medical school. Does this mean that behavior therapy should be practised by psychologists, rather than by psychiatrists? Such a question is not capable of being answered by someone who, like myself, is not intimately acquainted with the internal situation in the U. S. A.; in the U. K. the answer will probably be that both disciplines should work harmoniously together, each contributing, on a basis of absolute equality, what it is best qualified to contribute. Behavior therapy is only part, although often the most important part, of full psychiatric treatment; to cure a patient of his homosexuality, say, is not sufficient without a thoroughgoing program of follow-up services to teach him novel modes of adjustment, requiring social workers, and possibly psychiatrists. Drugs may be required, either independently or as part of the behavior therapy treatment; these can only be administered by a psychiatrist. Nothing can be gained, and much may be lost, by intransigence and hostility; in the public mind psychologists and psychiatrists are not clearly differentiated, and we are likely to be judged together according to the success or failure of our methods of treatment. There are not likely to be enough able people in either discipline to cope with a tenth of the likely demand; to dispute jurisdictional lines of demarcation at such a time is to be guilty of antisocial practices.

Simple behavior therapy methods could with advantage be taught to G.P.s; there is no reason why desensitization should not be practised by them, after a short course, even though more complex treatments would of course be reserved for more highly trained psychologists and psychiatrists. Altogether, the advent of these new methods obviously necessitates a complete rethinking of our organization of therapeutic and prophylactic activities, or training (both the *whom* and the *what)* and of examinations—can a person any longer claim to be a psychiatric specialist on the strength of having received an extensive training in methods which do not seem to have any therapeutic effects, and without having any competence in methods which have been shown to have such effects? Revolutions are never comfortable periods to live in; this is no different. However, the needs of the patient must come first, otherwise the oath of Hippocrates becomes the oath of Hypocrites! Clearly, all these issues require discussion, argument, and detailed investigation; it would be foolish of me to pretend to know the answers. Let us just remember that in the past few years there has been a drastic and dramatic change in the general position of psychiatric work; that we can no longer believe in the efficacy of psychotherapy or psychoanalysis, and that instead we now have strong evidence for the efficacy of new short-term methods of treatment under the general label of behavior therapy. These are the facts; how they are digested is a different problem which will differ in different countries, and whose solutions, too, will not necessarily be the same in the U. S. A., say, as in the U. K. What we cannot and must not do is to disregard these new findings and advances, and retire into the empty shell of our pristine inefficacy.

REFERENCES

Ayllon, T., and Azrin, N. (1968): *The Token Economy*. N. York: Wiley.

Bandura, A. (1969): *Principles of Behavior Modification*. N. York: Holt.

Cooper, J. E., Gelder, M. G., and Marks, I. M. (1965): Results of behaviour therapy in 77 psychiatric patients. *Brit. Med. J.,* 1, 1222-1225.

Eysenck, H. J. (1952): The effects of psychotherapy: an evaluation. *J. consult. Psychol.,* 16, 319-324.

Eysenck, H. J. (1958): Personality Tests: 1950- 1955. In: *Recent Progress in Psychiatry*. London: J & A Churchill. (Ed. G.W.T.H. Fleming).

Eysenck, H. J. (1959): Learning theory and behaviour therapy. *J. ment. Sci.,* 105, 61-75.

Eysenck, H. J. (1960): The effects of psychotherapy, in *Handbook of Abnormal Psychology*. Ed. H. J. Eysenck. London: Pitmans.

Eysenck, H. J. (1963): Beahviour Therapy, spontaneous remission and transference in neurotics. *Amer. J. Psychiat.,* 119, 867-871.
Eysenck, H. J. (Ed.) (1964): *Experiments in Behaviour Therapy.* Oxford: Pergamon Press.
Eysenck, H. J. (1967): *The Biological Basis of Personality.* Springfield: C. C. Thomas.
Eysenck, H. J. (1969): *The Effects of Psychotherapy.* N. York: Science House Inc.
Eysenck, H. J. (1970): Behaviour therapy and its critics. *J. Behav. Ther. & Exp. Psychiat.,* 1, 5-15.
Friess, C., and Nelson, M. J. (1942): Psychoneurotics five years later. *Amer. J. Medical Science,* 203, 539-558.
Gelder, M., Marks, I., and Wolfe, H. (1967): Desensitization and psychotherapy in the treatment of phobic states. *Brit. J. Psychiatry,* 113, 53-73.
Gillan, P. (1970): Behaviour therapy and psychotherapy: A comparative investigation. (In preparation).
Humphrey, J. (1966): Behaviour therapy with children: An experimental evaluation. Ph.D. Thesis. Univ. of London, 1966.
Imber, S. (1968): A ten-year follow-up of treated psychiatric outpatients. In: Lesse, S. (1968) (Ed.) *An evaluation of the results of the Psychotherapies.* Springfield: Thomas.
Krasner, L. (1962): The therapist as a social reinforcement machine, In: *Research in Psychotherapy,* APA.
Lang, P. J. (1969): The on-line computer in behaviour therapy research. *Am. Psychol.,* 24, 236.
Marks, I., and Gelder, M. (1965): A controlled retrospective study of behaviour therapy in phobic patients. *Br. J. Psychiat.,* 111, 561-573.
Marks, I., and Gelder, M. (1966): Severe agoraphobia. A controlled prospective trial of behaviour therapy. *Brit. J. Psychiatry,* 112, 309-320.
Marks, I. M., and Gelder, M. G. (1968): Different ages of onset in varieties of phobia. *Amer. J. Psychiatry,* 123, 218-221.
Marks, I. M., and Gelder, M. G. (1968): Controlled trials in behaviour therapy, in R. Porter (Ed.) *The Role of Learning in Psychotherapy.* London: J. & A. Churchill.
Marks, I. M., Gelder, M. G., and Edwards, G. (1968): Hypnosis and desensitization for phobias: a controlled prospective trial. *Br. J. Psychiatry,* 14, 1263.
Martin, I., Marks, I., and Gelder, M. (1969): Conditioned eyelid responses in phobic patients. *Beh. Res. & Therap.,* 7, 115-124.
Rachman, S. (1971): *The Effects of Psychotherapy.* To appear.
Rachman, S. (1965): Studies in desensitization: I. The separate effects of relaxation and desensitization. *Behav. Res. & Therapy,* 3, 245-252.
Rachman, S., and Teasdale, J. (1969): *Aversion Therapy and Behaviour Disorders.* London: Routledge & Kegan Paul.
Stevenson, I. (1961): Processes of "spontaneous" recovery from the psychoneuroses. *Amer. J. Psychiat.,* 117, 1057-1064.
Thompson, I. G. and Rathod, N. H. (1968): Aversion therapy for heroin dependence. *Lancet,* 17, 382.
Truax, C., and Carkhuff, R. (1967): *Toward Effective Counseling and Psychotherapy.* Chicago: Aldine Press.
Ullmann, L., and Krasner, L. (1969): *A Psychological Approach to Abnormal Behavior.* New Jersey: Prentice-Hall.

Wolpe, J. (1958): *Psychotherapy by Reciprocal Inhibition.* Stanford: Stanford Univ. Press.

Zubin, J., Eron, L. D., and Schumer, F. (1965): *An Experimental Approach to Projective Techniques.* New York: Wiley.

Part IV
Prevention

PREVENTION

Prevention is aimed at reducing the incidence of mental problems and breakdowns (primary prevention), preventing incipient problems from becoming worse (secondary prevention), and stabilizing people who have had an emotional disorder, received treatment, and are now back in the community (tertiary prevention). A typical method of accomplishing this is through consultation with social agencies and institutions regarding the "mental health atmosphere" of the agency, determining practices within the organization that lead to poor mental health, and identifying individuals with potentials for emotional disorder and then assisting administrators and staff in dealing with these problems. Agencies often chosen for consultation are those which are believed to have particularly important influences on the mental health of individuals, such as the schools, police, and welfare. Other methods include early identification of incipient emotional disturbance (e.g., students who are experiencing stress or unhappiness in the school situation are seen by the school psychologist to determine the nature and seriousness of the problems), follow-up of people who have shown emotional disturbance, and crisis intervention. Crisis intervention assumes that help at critical points in a person's life will prevent emotional breakdown.

Advocates of prevention see it as crucial in dealing with mental health on a community basis. Preventative approaches will reduce the number of people who need direct services and provide the only means by which limited mental health manpower can deal with the pervasive problems in the mental health field.

Those who oppose prevention do so for a variety of reasons. Some believe that preventative approaches are not effective. For example, consultation with a social agency rarely results in the agency changing its policies or procedures in the interests of good mental health. Crisis intervention deals with one or several crises in the life of an individual whose life pattern is a series of crises. There may be insufficient knowledge about emotional development and distrubance to know how to achieve primary prevention. These opponents believe that we are only expert in the giving of direct services and that by concentrating on preventative approaches we fritter away our scarce mental health manpower. Another reason for opposing preventative approaches is the belief that these lead the mental health worker to fragment services and give up professional responsibility. For example, in doing consultation, the consultant is not responsible for the carrying out of the advice and suggestions he makes and implementation is usually in the hands of a variety of other people who may be unable or unwilling to do what the consultant thinks is necessary. Also, some opponents believe that preventative approaches such as methods of early identification of emotional problems or follow-up often involve an invasion of privacy.

Dr. Henry Grunebaum and Dr. Gerald Caplan have been associates at The Laboratory of Community Psychiatry at Harvard Medical School. Dr. Caplan is director of the laboratory and Dr. Grunebaum currently is Director, Family and Child Development Study, Harvard Medical School. Dr. Caplan has played a leading role in the United States in developing preventative programs in community mental health. He has pioneered a carefully defined and differentiated method of mental health consultation. Dr. Grunebaum has been active in developing training programs in community psychiatry. In the article that follows, Dr. Grunebaum and Dr. Caplan present a conceptual framework for primary prevention and give examples of its applications.

Dr. Elaine Cumming is Professor and Chairman, Department of Anthropology and Sociology, University of Victoria, British Columbia, Canada. Formerly she was Director, Mental Health Research Unit of the New York State Department of Mental Hygiene, and Adjunct Professor of Sociology at the State University at Albany. She is well known for her research into various aspects of social deviance and social control. Dr. Cumming presents a critical view of primary prevention.

PERSPECTIVES ON PRIMARY PREVENTION: A REVIEW*

Gerald Caplan and Henry Grunebaum

In recent years psychiatrists have come to realize that psychological maldevelopment, maladaptation, and illness are so prevalent that treatment of established cases can never be expected to deal adequately with more than a fraction of the cases which occur. Therefore, one must consider how to reduce the incidence of mental illness, as well as to promote mental health. Primary prevention is that preventive effort which is concerned with studying the population-wide patterns of forces influencing the lives of people in order to learn how to reduce the risk of mental disorder.

Although we currently have little definite knowledge of the specific factors which are etiologic in specific mental diseases, there exists a body of plausible assumptions about various factors which may be significant in primary prevention. Some of these assumptions are based on experiments on human beings and animals, others are inferred from theory. Some are based upon experiences in psychotherapy, psychoanalysis, and clinical research. Others are derived from epidemiological studies which demonstrate the existence of different sets of conditions in communities which have high rates of mental disorder, as contrasted with those which have low rates.

* Reprinted from *Archives of General Psychiatry*, Vol. 17, Sept. 1967, with permission of authors and editor.

TYPES OF PREVENTION

Preventive psychiatry can be considered under three main headings.

Primary Prevention aims at reducing the incidence of new cases of mental disorder and disability in a population. Efforts are focused both on modifying the environment and strengthening individual capacities to cope with situations. We will discuss primary prevention in this paper, and it can best be understood if secondary and tertiary prevention are also briefly described.

Secondary Prevention aims at reducing the duration of cases of mental disorder which will inevitably occur in spite of the programs of primary prevention. By shortening the duration of existing cases, the prevalence of mental disorder in the community is reduced. This may be accomplished by organizing case-finding, diagnostic, and remedial services so that mental disorders are detected early and are dealt with efficiently and effectively.

Tertiary Prevention aims at reducing the community rate of residual defect which is often a sequel to acute mental illness. It seeks to ensure that people who have recovered from mental disorder will be hampered as little as possible by their past difficulties in returning to full participation in the occupational and social life of the community. Alienation of the patient from work, family, and social groups during and after mental illness may be diminished by programs to rehabilitate ex-patients, so that symptom reduction will be complemented by the recovery of old occupational and social skills or the acquisition of new ones.

All three preventive effects focus on groups within the total population and seek to reduce the community rates of mental disorder and its effects. This is the new approach advocated in 1963 by the late President Kennedy. It contrasts with an approach which provides therapists and institutions with responsibilities restricted to their individual patients. There are now increasing efforts to take into account those individuals who define themselves as patients and seek assistance, those who do not avail themselves of help yet who suffer from mental illness, and those who are currently healthy.

In order to effect prevention there will, of necessity, have to be planned programs so that the deployment of specialized resources will be related to appropriate aims; and evaluation of effectiveness will have to be built into the programs from the outset. Mental health programs will have to be coordinated with other programs in the community which influence the psychological life conditions of its citizens. Clearly community planning, organization, and coordination are fundamental elements in effecting preventive psychiatry. Thus the key factors which influence mental health in the community must be delineated in the areas of economics, politics, public health, religion, welfare, and education, to name a few. It will be obvious that the lines between the roles of psychiatrist, social planner, and social activist will often not be clear. Each individual will have to decide for himself which of these tasks he will undertake at any given time, just as he must decide to what extent to focus his efforts on individuals or groups, research or education. Insofar as possible, primary prevention is the most desirable and potentially most effective approach to a solution of the problem of mental disorder in our communities. At the present, however, primary prevention is clearly more a hope than a reality.

PRIMARY PREVENTION

In order to deal systematically with primary prevention, the following conceptual framework will be used to order the data. According to this model, the rate of mental disorder in a community is related to the interaction of both long-term and short-term factors which impinge on adaptive capacities of its members. However, the individual person is not merely the passive recipient of what the environment provides, but actively organizes his environment to obtain what he may need. Any individual's ability to cope with his environment will, of course, vary over the long and short term. Similarly, the human environment varies widely in its richness, organization, and comprehensibility. We may call those environmental factors which impinge on the individual *resources*, if it is clear that we are not merely interested in the quantity of a resource but also in its organization, timing, duration, quality, and other relevant variables. (The word "resource" is not entirely satisfactory, and "supplies" and "opportunities" are possible alternatives.)

Over the long term, the likelihood of psychological dysfunction is increased if specified basic resources are not adequately provided for the population; these resources may be classified as physical, psychological, and sociocultural. A program of primary prevention will seek to evaluate these resources and ensure their optimal provision in the population.

The *short-term* focus of this preventive model is on the pattern of adaptation to developmental and situational life crises. It appears likely that the direction of a person's psychological development throughout life, whether toward mental health or disorder, is most sensitive to influence at times of crisis. These crises represent transition points, at each of which the person may move nearer or further away from adaptive patterns of functioning. Primary preventive efforts are often directed toward modifying the field of forces at times of crisis in the belief that efforts may be more effectively and more efficiently applied at these times.

NATURE OF LONG-TERM RESOURCES

Physical resources include food, shelter, adequate living space,[1] sensory stimulation,[2] and opportunities for exercise, sleeping,[3] dreaming,[4] etc. These are necessary for growth and development, and for the maintenance of the bodily health upon which mental health is dependent. Protection is necessary from bodily damage, such as that by radiation, microorganisms, trauma, or chemical poisons, both before and after birth.

Psychosocial resources include the stimulation of a person's intellectual and emotional development through personal interaction with significant others.

These include members of his family, peers, and other persons in school, church, and work. In face-to-face interchanges the person satisfies his needs for love and affection, limitation and control, and participation in joint activity which provides opportunities for identification and identity formation. Inadequate provision of psychosocial resources may be conducive to mental disorder for example, if there is a disorder in the relationships with parents, or if satisfactory relationships are interrupted through illness, death, or departure.

Sociocultural resources include those influences on personality development and functioning which are exerted by the social structure of community and culture. The expectations by others of a person's behavior have a profound influence on psychological development and the growth of self-esteem. Man's place in the structure of his society is determined by others to a large extent, and they prescribe his path in life to a considerable degree. If a person happens to be born into an advantaged group in a stable society, his social roles and their expected changes over a lifetime will tend to provide him with adequate opportunities for healthy personality development. If, on the other hand, he belongs to a disadvantaged minority, suffers from economic deprivation,[5] or is a member of an unstable society, as Leighton[6] has shown, he may find his progress blocked and he may be deprived of opportunity and challenge. This may have an adverse effect on his mental health. Calhoun[1] has demonstrated the deleterious effects of overcrowding on the laboratory animal, and it may well be the case that for psychological health there is an optimal human population in any given area, just as there is an optimal population for a given level of food supplies.

IMPROVING THE PROVISION OF LONG-TERM RESOURCES

Primary prevention involves studying the provision of resources in a population and attempting to improve the situation when necessary—usually by modifying community-wide practices through changing laws, regulations, administrative patterns, or wide-spread values and attitudes. The following examples are illustrative.

Physical or Nonhuman Resources. Examples of host factors which may be influenced to prevent the development of mental disorder include efforts to prevent prematurity, which adversely influences intellectual development; to provide appropriate nutrition for children with genetic defects, such as phenylketonuria;[7] and the provision of iodinated salt in areas where iodine supplies may be inadequate, as to prevent the endemic cretinism which causes mental retardation.[8] Another example is the prevention of psychosis due to the pellagra caused by vitamin B deficiency. This has been much reduced in the southern part of the United States by social policies and community education programs which have fostered changes in the food habits and food supplies of the population.[9] The environment, on the other hand, may provide easy access to poisons: for example, lead poisoning in slum children from eating lead paint off decaying woodwork is not uncommon.[10] This could be prevented by laws requiring landlords to replace old lead-containing paint with modern lead-free varieties.

The effect of inadequate environmental stimulation and its consequent effect on cognitive development is at present under intensive investigation. Already, however, the work of Hess[11] and Deutsch[12] is sufficient to indicate the importance of the early perceptual experiences of the child for later intellectual development. It has been found that the cognitive environment of severely deprived groups impairs later learning.[13,14] Efforts at cognitive enrichment for pre-school children through education, as in Operation Headstart (Office of Economic Opportunity, Washington, DC), are being undertaken, and evaluations of such programs are urgently needed.

In a different area, it is found that the sensory deprivations or distortions experienced by patients undergoing cataract operations[15] or cardiac surgery[16] can cause a transient psychosis which may be prevented by appropriate intervention. These examples would appear to imply strongly that certain aspects of the physical environment have direct psychological consequences of significance to mental health.

Psychosocial Resources. Under this heading we will comment upon those factors which impinge on an individual in his face-to-face interchanges with others. These include the stimulation of an individual's intellectual and emotional development through personal interaction with significant people in his family, peer group, and people in authority.

A central issue here is the maintenance of a healthy family environment. For instance, legislators and administrators who plan manpower distribution should be influenced to ensure that fathers be given work opportunities in the localities where their families live. Employment regulations concerning pregnant women and mothers of young children should allow them time off to care for their children. In some countries, graduated family allowances encourage mothers of young children to stay at home with them. Divorce laws and legal practices relating to custody of children are an important field for the consultative services of the psychiatrist. In Denmark, for instance, a mental health specialist is consulted whenever a couple with children seeks a divorce, and his advice influences court decisions on custody and visiting.

Illness, hospitalization, or death of the mother are common problems often leading to fragmentation of the family; the children are separated and sent to unstable placements with relatives or to foster homes and residential institutions. For instance, Rice[17] found in a study of the children of women who were hospitalized for psychosis, that no professional assistance in arranging care for the children was sought or offered in these cases, and that the children experienced many placements at the very time when they needed extra emotional support.

The works of Spitz,[18] Bowlby,[19] and Provence and Lipton[20] have demonstrated the importance of adequate mothering and the deleterious effects of impersonal institutions on child development. Yet it is not institutions qua institutions which are harmful. Skeels[21] has recently reported a remarkable 20-year follow-up of two matched groups of orphans, one of which was raised in an impersonal institution and the other in a home for the mentally retarded, where the children received much attention and stimulation prior to adoption. The second group of children was functioning in the community as adults while the first group remained, with one exception, institutionalized. The human and financial costs of these two types of institutions differ strikingly; this study points out again that institutions need not have adverse effects, but can, under certain conditions, irreversibly damage development. The care of children by Aid to Dependent Children[22] and those in public institutions are striking instances where psychiatric knowledge[23,24] is sufficiently expert to provide adequate guidelines for planning, yet where public policy lags tragically behind what is known.[25] A preventive program would seek to ensure provision by the community of both an adequate homemaker service, so that families could be kept together in their own homes as much as possible, and the provision of adequate institutions when necessary.

The effect of loss of the mother when a child is hospitalized has been recently reviewed by Mason.[26] This remains a classical example of the failure to provide for essential psychosocial needs, and it could be avoided by regulations promoting daily visiting of hospitalized children by their parents, modification of hospital structure and functioning to allow mothers to stay with and help nurse their children (which might alleviate in small part the shortage of personnel), changes in the professional practice of pediatrics as advocated by Prugh,[24] and efforts to treat sick children at home rather than in hospital as much as possible.

The maintenance of family ties is not only important

in childhood but throughout life, particularly in old age. Significant developments in present-day urban life are the relative increase in the number of the aged due to improvements in general health care, and the difficulty of maintaining regular contact between the older and younger generations. This is partly caused by policies and the attitudes of both generations. Understanding psychological factors might influence city planners to provide more large apartments, especially in housing projects, so that grandparents need not be pushed out of the family home. Planners, on the other hand, could be counseled to build special housing for the aged in relatively small units spread throughout the community, so that old people can live near and maintain contact with their children and grandchildren.

One of the programs of the antipoverty effort, "Foster Grandparents" (Older Persons Program, Office of Economic Opportunity, Washington, D.C.), has been to provide foster grandparents for poor children. In this instance, children and old people are brought together who are not related by blood but by geographical proximity. These programs have seemed beneficial to both sets of participants and need not be limited to the poor. It may be possible to combat the attitudes of rejection of the aged by programs of public education to help younger people understand the problems and potentials of their parents and grandparents in much the same way that we try to increase their understanding of children.

Sociocultural Resources. The most obvious example of ensuring the provision of sociocultural resources in efforts at primary prevention is that of influencing the educational system. The role of psychiatrists in offering consultation to educators to help them improve the psychological atmosphere of the school is well-known. It is also true that psychiatrists are increasingly becoming involved in the social and educational environment of colleges and universities,[27] and a recent report by the Group for the Advancement of Psychiatry entitled "Sex and the College Student,"[28] illustrates an attempt to inform college administrators about psychological issues of direct relevance to them.

Barger[29] has studied the epidemiology of failure to

graduate in a university community. He delineated groups of students at special risk, discovered times of increased incidence of breakdown, and then instituted social action, including anticipatory orientation sessions for freshmen, consultation to caregivers such as chaplains, and specially supportive dormitory arrangements for individuals identified as being at risk. The effectiveness of this program is being studied now.

Another example is Upward Bound (Community Action Program, Office of Economic Opportunity, Washington, DC), a preventive program which has recently been initiated in a metropolitan slum. In this area the scholastic levels of many young people who leave high school were no longer sufficient to the demands of the labor market because of rapid technological advances leading to diminished needs for unskilled labor. The result was rising unemployment among young people with inadequate education, which had obvious effects on their psychological health that led to frustration, depression, and tendencies to rebel against the social order which they felt was rejecting them. The neighborhood had an increased incidence of delinquency, alcoholism, drug addiction, illegitimate pregnancies, abortion, and venereal disease—all signs of social disorganization. Attempts to deal with these problems by traditional casework and remedial psychiatric practices had about as much effect as trying to bail out a flooded room with a small bucket while the water continued to pour in from a burst pipe. Now, a new preventive service has been instituted which attempts to handle the problems at their sources. A systematic program of improving the educational offerings of the school system in that neighborhood has been instituted. Extra teachers of high caliber were hired, and more modern educational techniques were instituted. At the same time, efforts at raising the levels of aspiration of the students and their families were begun by involving the entire community in an adult educational campaign in an attempt to increase the motivation of the students to stay at school and to study as hard as students in middle-class school districts, with the hope and the confidence that the technologically advanced labor market will be open to them. Here again, a plausible program has been initiated, but an evaluation of the results has not been reported.

The sociocultural needs of the aged population may be met by modifying retirement laws and regulations so that older people who retain their capacities are not forced to retire suddenly and prematurely and may be offered part-time or light-work opportunities as their powers diminish. Old age assistance and retirement pensions could take up the slack in income as earning capacity is reduced by age if regulations did not penalize a person for working. In certain cases, at present, the lowered earning capacity of older people means that their income may be less if they work than if they were entirely unemployed and drawing full welfare assistance. Studies, such as that in progress at Harvard Medical School's Laboratory of Community Psychiatry under McEwan and Sheldon are urgently needed so that retirement can be planned in terms of individual needs and capacities, and so that those who are vulnerable to postretirement difficulties may be identified and assisted.

Social isolation is a potent factor in promoting mental disorders in the aged.[30] A preventive program would foster the provision of social and recreational facilities, administered in a way to stimulate the activity and independence of the aged rather than permitting them to become the passive recipients of care. In preparation for retirement, health education programs aimed at the middle-aged population can use anticipatory guidance, so that people can face in advance the implications of old age and see this period as one in which they will be expected and encouraged to remain interested in the social, political, welfare, and recreational life of their community, and productively active in formal work, service, or in sheltered occupations.

In all examples of these kinds, it is necessary to identify the physical, psychosocial, or sociocultural factors at work in the community, and to modify social policy. Education of professional or lay groups and efforts at influencing legislators and administrators to modify laws, regulations, and policies may be necessary. These efforts are often successful, and psychiatrists and psychologists have been influential in changing policies in such institutions as industry[31, 32] and the Army.[33] Thus, the Army has found that treating neuropsychiatric casualties as close to the front lines as possible has led to a much higher salvage rate than was the case when they were treated far from their unit.

It is worth emphasizing that this is not government by psychiatrists. Legislators and administrators will perforce take into consideration many economic, social, and political issues before making their decisions. Primary prevention, however, involves the psychiatrist as a participant in social planning and social action, so that those who govern may take into account the mental health needs of their populations. It is to be hoped that if these are infringed upon, it is done with some knowledge and consideration of the consequences. For example, the psychiatrist may point out that an urban relocation program is likely to have an adverse effect on the aged inhabitants of a condemned area. Fried,[34] in particular, has demonstrated the results of an ill-concerned urban renewal program on the inhabitants of a lower-class but highly organized community. Nevertheless, the economy of the city may demand that the slum be torn down and replaced by modern apartment houses. The legislators, who have been informed of the psychological sequelae of renewal, may then feel obligated to provide extra social work and home nursing service to the old people, to give them special help in handling their relocation difficulties. According to communications from a Visiting Nurses Association, this did in fact occur in the city under discussion. Legislators may also be inclined to solicit the advice of psychiatrists in planning other measures to cushion the blow, such as making provision for ethnic and extended family groups to be rehoused near each other and near the places where their old social and recreational agencies have been relocated.

SHORT-TERM OR CRISIS FACTORS

Up to this point we have discussed the preventive psychiatric implications of impairments or inadequacies of the host-environment interaction; this interaction, long-term in duration, affects the steady process of psychological development. Sometimes, however, individuals face immediate problems from whch they cannot escape, and which are beyond their capacities to solve. This results in states of temporary disequilibrium in the relatively smooth trajectory of development. These emotionally significant turning points, or crises,[35] are short periods usually marked by psychological upsets.

Crisis theory has been derived from a series of research projects carried out over the past 15 years. Some typical examples are the crisis of bereavement,[36,37] the reactions of parents to the birth of a normal or of a premature child,[38,39] and the crisis of surgery.[40] There are recent studies of the crises experienced by Peace Corps volunteers exposed to unexpected cultural problems in their overseas assignments,[41] and by engaged and newly married couples in dealing with the ordinary upsets of early married life.[42] Clinical work suggests that deterioration of mental health often occurs following such crises; and it appears that during the crisis significant psychological changes must occur. On the other hand, healthy coping has also been described, such as in the work of Silber et al.[43,44] with competent adolescents. Findings to date point to the potential value of studying the psychological processes which take place during crises in order to find leverage points for improving the outcome. Parad's[45] book of readings covers many aspects of clinical and investigative work in this field.

The terminology in the field is unsettled; thus, the word "crisis" was originally used by Lindemann and Caplan to refer to personal reaction after such traumatic events as sudden bereavement or the birth of a premature child. Erikson, on the other hand, uses the same word to refer to a series of normal developmental steps such as those of puberty or menopause. Crisis may thus be employed to refer to both normal and unusual transitions which necessitate specific tasks of interpersonal and intrapsychic readjustment. Recently Rapoport,[46] who has studied couples through engagement, honeymoon, and early marriage, has called attention to the social aspects of this transition by calling it a "critical role transition."[46] On the other hand, Parkes (unpublished), using an approach influenced by Kurt Lewin, suggests using the term "change in life space." He criticizes the word "crisis" as referring to the emotional results of the transition which may in fact be absent, as in a delayed grief reaction. In the interests of simplicity we will continue to employ the term "crisis," recognizing that certain examples are marked by society for recognition through ritual and may be called "critical role transitions." Others are due to alteration in the life space, while yet others are due to biological maturation. All of these junction points involve change in role as well as interpsychic and intrapsychic balance; the differentiation is one of emphasis.

Crisis may be due to either internal or external changes necessitating adaptation. The internal changes may be developmental or due to illness or trauma, while the external changes involve (a) the loss of a significant person or source of need satisfaction, (b) the threat of loss, or (c) a challenge which threatens to overtax adaptive capacities. This list strikingly resembles the causes of neurosis delineated by Freud,[47] who in 1912 mentioned (1) frustration due to loss of an object, (2) inability to adapt to a challenge such as marriage, (3) inhibition in development, and (4) biologic maturation.

During crisis the individual's usual pattern of functioning becomes disorganized. He feels anxious, and thought processes are often confused and ineffective. Particularly evident is a preoccupation with the problem which precipitated the upset, and memories of similar problems from the past. Feelings of frustration and helplessness are common. Crises usually last for a period of up to four to six weeks. By the end of that time the anxiety usually diminishes, and the person returns to a steady psychological and physiological state as he works out a solution. It is of interest that recent investigations demonstrate specific biochemical concomitants of specific phases of emotional crisis.[48] The problem may be dealt with in an adaptive way by realistic modification of the environment and by intrapsychic readjustments. On the other hand, the solution may be (1) postponed, as in delayed grief; (2) maladaptive; or (3) development of psychiatric symptoms. It is believed that the methods of crisis resolution used by the individual—whether healthy or maladaptive—will become henceforward a part of his coping repertoire and may be used in dealing with future problems. Thus the individual may emerge from the crisis with increased adaptive capacities and confidence in his ability to tolerate stress and to cope. On the other hand, he may emerge with lower adaptive capacities and a greater vulnerability to mental disorder. Therefore, we can say that crises represent mental health turning points. The individual will be helped or hindered in finding a healthy outcome by his family and friends. Work has recently suggested that conjoint family interviews at times of crisis offer insight into the degree to which the family is helping the person toward an adaptive or maladaptive solution.[49] He may also be helped by community caregivers, such as doctors, lawyers, teachers, clergymen, and social workers. This is of importance, because a person in crisis both feels a greater need for help than when he is in his usual psychological state, and *is usually more easily influenced* during this period than at other times.[49] He is in unstable equilibrium. A crisis, therefore, represents a leverage point; this means that assistance may produce a greater effect if focused on people at times of crisis than during periods of stable equilibrium, and an opportunity is thus available to maximize the potential of our scarce mental health specialists.

APPLICATIONS OF CRISIS THEORY

Preventive psychiatric efforts, based on studies of

crisis, have been attempted and are focused on two broad goals.

Reducing Severity of Crises

It is not possible to prevent crises altogether. Temporarily unsurmountable problems are an inevitable aspect of life; and there will always be unexpected and stressful situations to be faced, such as illness, death, accidents, and operations. Normal development implies coping with change. Even if it were possible to avoid all stress and challenge, we would not wish to do so; *The Happy Prince* by Oscar Wilde illustrates the grief that befalls one who attempts to avoid all the sadness consequent to life. The successful mastery of challenge provides the opportunity for personality growth and enrichment, as Zetzel[50] pointed out recently in a paper on the problems that individuals who have never developed the capacity for dealing with grief and depression must face.

It does appear, however, that if stress can be kept within tolerable bounds, the crisis will be less intense and there will be a better chance of healthy adaptive responses. It may be useful to study the living conditions of the community in order to identify those circumstances which precipitate crisis in significant numbers of the population, and to modify those circumstances, if possible, so that their impact is reduced.

For example, it was found in a midwestern community[51] that many young married couples with several children were seeking assistance from social agencies, ministers, and physicians because of disturbance in their children or dissatisfaction with their marriage. Clinical and epidemiological investigation turned up the pertinent fact that a significant number of these couples had married because of premarital pregnancy. When the pregnancy was first discovered, they had consulted their ministers, priests, or physicians, and these caregivers had encouraged them to marry. When the later consequences of these marriages were discussed with the persons who had been consulted at the time of crisis, they realized that a deeper review of the problem of pre-marital pregnancy and due consideration of alternative solutions might have been more useful in the long run. The effects of this changed approach to a crisis situation are now under study. It may be added that one of the counselors, a priest, had come to the same conclusion as the psychiatrist independently on the basis of his own experience.

Services to Foster Healthy Crisis-Coping

It has already been stated that the outcome of a crisis is influenced by the quality of help which the individual receives from family, friends, and community caregivers in trying to work out a new adaptation. The psychiatrist is part of this potentially helpful influence network. Since he cannot personally help large numbers of people in crisis, his major impact can only come from indirect action, which may take the following paths.

Ensuring That Communities Provide Professional Help During Crisis. In order for professionals to help an individual in crisis, it is necessary for them to understand the nature of crisis reactions and to have the necessary therapeutic skill. In addition, administration policy must be such that they are immediately available to offer help during relatively short periods of crisis disequilibrium when critical choices of coping pattern are being made. The increased desire for help during crisis will impel the person to ask for assistance; but, unless he can gain access to the agency and the helper during the crisis period itself—a period no longer than a few weeks in duration—he will have to cope unaided.

This situation presents no problem in many types of crises, because the predicament itself is so clearly a life emergency that immediate contact with a community agency or caregiving professional is mandatory: for example, a surgical emergency, a road accident, or a death in the family. In many other instances, however, the predicament, apart from the psychological crisis, is not an obvious emergency: examples are the crises of adolescence, early marriage, change of jobs, entrance into nursery school, or retirement. In these cases the individual or his family must reach out for help from a health, welfare, education, or religious agency. Unfortunately, many of these agencies are not prepared to handle new cases quickly. They have long waiting lists, and their clientele are usually chronic cases involving treatment long in duration but not necessarily immediately available. Such agencies usually conceive an "emergency case" as one of obvious and dramatic severity, and only such cases are likely to be given priority on waiting lists. Crisis upsets are often not dramatic despite their importance, and therefore would not be given priority. Agency policy should attempt to shorten and abolish waiting lists, and staff should be available for immediate help. Centers for the prevention of suicide, available 24 hours a day, are an example in this direction,[52] although their effectiveness over time must be studied. Reeducation of staff may be necessary to accomplish these changes.

A survey of commonly occurring crises may disclose that some fall outside the sphere of current agency operations. If this is the case, it may be necessary to attempt to influence the community planning and governing bodies either to assign new jurisdictions to old agencies, or to establish new agencies to cover areas of unmet need. A common example of a lacuna in agency practice is the absence of adequate home-maker services in many communities. Their provision would ensure that families facing the temporary absence of mothers may be kept together in their homes, thus ameliorating the stress of this crisis.[53] In many communities no agencies are available to assist widows or parents who are divorced. The Cruse clubs[54] in England and Parents Without Partners[55] in this country have grown up in recent years as a response to these problems. The development of such community initiatives should clearly be encouraged. On the other hand, in many rural areas traditional family and child welfare agencies are completely absent; their provision must be a major goal of those involved in the primary prevention of mental disorder.[56]

Preventive   Intervention   With   Individuals   in Crisis. Klein and Lindemann,[57] Waldfogel and Gardner,[58] and Rapoport[46] have discussed techniques of preventive intervention by mental health specialists during the period of disorganization of a crisis in an individual and his family. Parad[59] has recently surveyed the efforts of a number of projects concerned with various styles of time-limited crisis intervention to individuals and families. Unpublished studies at the Laboratory of Community Psychiatry of Harvard Medical School confirm this approach and suggest the importance of the following methodogical points.

Timing.

The most economic utilization of professional efforts is achieved by repeated visits at short intervals during the four to six week period of the crisis rather than by interviews at weekly intervals for many months.

Family Orientation.

Intervention should support the integrity of the family in its own home if possible, and prevent its fragmentation in order to conserve its capacity to support the family member who is most directly affected by the crisis. Thus, if a parent is absent or deceased, a replacement from within the family or by a homemaker should be obtained. Families can be helped to share the painful affect consequent to the crisis and comfort and support each other, as well as assist each other in household tasks. To these ends, interviews in the home with couples and whole families may be useful.

Avoiding Dependency.

Individuals in crisis are more dependent; however, long-term dependency does not appear to be fostered by active intervention during crises. In fact, the more help given during the crisis, the more independent are the clients when the crisis has been resolved. Undue dependency is also avoided by dealing with current realities rather than exploring the antecedents of the problem.

Fostering Mastery.

The focus of crisis-oriented intervention is to enable the individual to master the problem by confronting it, despite the unpleasant affect it arouses, and the frustration of an unknown outcome. The individual requires all the information possible to deal effectively with the problem and to understand its predictable phases; so a useful model is the' one of education. Task-oriented activity is thus to be encouraged and hope maintained. An individual frequently releases tension associated with crisis by such nongoal-directed activities as redecorating a house, moving, or scapegoating a child; this wasteful activity has to be discouraged.

Outside Supports.

During the crisis period, the individual not only needs additional family support but the outside support of extended family, friends, clergy, and other agencies is most important. These are often not utilized for fear that asking for help is a sign of weakness. Clients can appropriately be reassured that this is not the case. It seems likely that nonprofessionals can often be most useful in offering support during a crisis, particularly if they themselves have experienced a similar one in the past.

Goals.

The goal of crisis intervention is to enable the individual to cope effectively with the current situation regardless of what past maladaptive experiences he may have had. The effort is thus to achieve an improvement in present functioning, rather a "cure." Since the focus of the work is on the final common path of going through the steps necessary to resolve the crisis rather than exploring its antecedents, it may not require specialized psychological knowledge or sophistication; nonprofessionals can thus be trained and supported in carrying it out.

Education of Caregivers. The caregiving professionals—doctors, nurses, clergymen, teachers, lawyers, etc.—are the major resource to whom people in crisis turn. To ensure that these caregivers attend to the mental health implications of the crisis and act skillfully, they must be appropriately educated in the necessary skills. They must learn enough about specific crises to know what psychological tasks are involved in ameliorating each, as well as what is within the range of healthy and unhealthy patterns of coping in order to identify and aid those individuals who are proceeding on a maladaptive course. For example, recent research[60] has shown that normal children experience a considerable degree of difficulty in going to elementary school, and it takes a surprisingly long time for them to adapt. Among others, Bower[61] has been interested in how we may aid children to better manage the transitions inherent in schooling.

Careful studies have shown that the premature birth of a child is a crisis for a family, and that physicians and nurses can be made aware that the pattern of the mother's initial adjustment to the situation may have a significant effect on her subsequent relationship to and care of her child.[62,63] Mothers who are coping poorly can be identified; for example, the mother who seems overly cheerful and unconcerned about the situation, who shows little curiosity about her baby's progress and about the meaning of prematurity, who visits him infrequently in the premature baby nursery, and who does not seek help from family members, friends, or professionals in dealing with the problems involved, indicates that on the whole she tends to evade or deny. A mother such as this can often be helped to recognize some of her realistic problems, and can be supported in admitting to consciousness and mastering her natural feelings of anxiety, guilt, and sadness. She can be encouraged to visit her baby regularly and learn how to understand and predict his progress by observing his behavior and getting relevant information about prematurity from the nurses. She can also be assisted to enlist the support of clergymen, public health nurses, and physicians as indicated, to help her with the problems which emerge.

Knowledge of the predictable emotional crises in the community can be communicated to the appropriate community caregivers by taking part in their preprofessional education or by participating in on-the-job training, as in postgraduate seminars for teachers, clergymen, or general practitioners. However, knowledge often lies fallow, as Mason has pointed out in a recent article. He noted the disparity between what is known about the adverse effects on children of separation from their parents during hospitalization, and the lag in pediatric practice and attitudes that still prevails.[26] This article illustrates how difficult it is to influence other professionals and organizations, and should lead to humility about our effectiveness. It also points up the need for studies which may enable us to be more successful in this task.

Mental Health Consultation. However well educated the community caregivers are with regard to crises, it is inevitable that they will encounter unexpected difficulties as they deal with emotional problems. In order to consolidate a program of preventive work by caregivers it is important to provide them with opportunities for consulting a mental health specialist. Various methods of consultation have been developed for use by mental health specialists in recent years.[64] For instance, in one city a mental health consultant goes for about two hours every week into each of the 20 health stations from which the nurses of the Public Health Department and the Visiting Nurse Association operate. Nurses who find themselves unable to understand particularly difficult cases or psychologically complicated problems in their patients are free to seek consultation in order to clarify the complexities. This enables them and their supervisors to work out improved ways of helping their patients.[35] Similar consultation programs exist in many communities, in schools, and in other community agencies.

Much work is necessary to devise and evaluate the appropriate techniques for consultation with different professions in their unique work situations. Although evaluation of the efficacy of consultation is just beginning, a study of consultation with nurses has recently been completed by Howe and Caplan (unpublished). It suggests that if issues emotionally relevant to the nurse are foci of the consultation, it is useful in the long run. However, space does not permit adequate coverage of this rapidly growing field; it deserves a review in its own right.

Education of Informal Caregivers. Individuals in crisis often turn for help not to professional caregivers, but to people who live or work near them, whom they have learned to know and respect. Such informal caregivers include neighbors, druggists, bartenders, hairdressers, industrial foremen, etc. They are chosen by people as confidants because of special personality gifts—capacity for empathy and understanding, and interest in their fellow men.

These informal caregivers exert a significant influence on the mental health of the population, and pose a major challenge for preventive psychiatry. How can we make contact with them, and how can we educate them so that they give wise counsel to those in crisis who seek them out? They have had no formal training, and we have had no hand in selecting them. Currently, pioneering efforts are being made to train and utilize indigenous workers in many places and in many programs. The work of Christmas,[65] Rieff[66] and Reissman,[67] and our own experiences[68] are examples.

Another way of reaching informal caregivers may be through mass media such as articles, radio, or TV. An example is an article entitled "Crisis in the Family,"[69] addressed to and hopefully read by those to whom people in crisis turn for help. It offers a series of guidelines or basic principles which may be useful in the helping process. Another example is illustrated by "Trouble in the Family," (Audio-Visual Center, National Educational Television Film Service) a television program which was recently honored by the American Psychiatric Association Strecker Award. A series of family therapy interviews conducted by Dr. Norman Paul was presented, with a commentary on the efforts of the family to improve their relationship with a problem child.

Personal Preparation for Healthy Crisis Coping Through Education. The effort here is to modify the content and methods of the education of children and youth so that skills are acquired for dealing adequately with unexpected and temporarily insoluble problems. An example is the attempt developed in Iowa by Ojemann[70] to improve the problem-solving capacities of children. The nature of American education, he observes, leads to what he calls "surface thinking," in which behavior in any situation is rather simply and automatically determined as a reaction to the overt manifestations of the problem. In place of this he advocates a "causal approach," in which the person learns to uncover the causes of the observed manifestations and then systematically works out a plan of action to deal with the most crucial of these causes. Ojemann has rewritten school textbooks and has trained teachers in methods of teaching causal thinking as an integral part of a normal school curriculum. The results were evaluated by comparing children taught along these lines with children from traditional classes; they clearly demonstrate that children taught the causal approach are better able to solve novel intellectual problems. They develop an increased capacity to persevere in the face of ambiguity, as well as an increased tolerance of frustration;[71] these are precisely the attributes which foster an improved capacity to deal adaptively with crisis. Biber[72] and others at the Bank Street School have been similarly interested in modifying the school experience to promote healthier adjustment and more successful problem solving by preschool and elementary school children.

Another approach is that of Kurt Hahn[73] and the Outward Bound movement in Britain, a program which was one of the forerunners of the Peace Corps. This program attempts character building experiential education for adolescents and young adults. The students are exposed to situations of natural hazard, such as climbing mountains or ocean sailing—or, in the Peace Corps, physical deprivation and cultural conflict. The stress is graduated to be just beyond the usual capacity of the student. He experiences an induced crisis, but is then provided with adult support and guidance in working his way to a healthy adaptation. This, it seems likely, will lead to a strengthening and maturing of his personality, with increased independence and awareness of his own capacities and improved skills in making use of the help of others.

These apparently relatively successful attempts point to the possibility of modifying our educational system on a wide population basis to improve the potential of students to master life crises. It is a field in which collaboration of psychiatrists with educators may yield important results in the future.

Anticipatory Guidance.   Here the effort is to prepare an individual for an impending crisis. An example is discussed in a recent study by Janis, of Yale,[74] which shows that among patients awaiting operation in a surgical ward, it is possible to predict which ones will have the least difficult postoperative psychological adjustment. Patients who are moderately worried about the operation and ask a lot of questions about the pain and discomfort ahead adapt more easily afterwards than those who seem unusually cheerful and express unconcern about the impending stress. The study suggests that if a person facing a crisis knows ahead of time what he must cope with and begins to master it, he will be better prepared psychologically to handle the stress when the situation is upon him. Janis recommends, on the basis of careful studies of postoperative patients, that patients awaiting operation should be given a sort of "emotional inoculation," wherein they are told in some detail what is likely to happen. Similarly, work in the Anesthesiology Department of the Massachusetts General Hospital[75] demonstrates that it is possible to reduce the postoperative narcotic requirements by approximately half through preoperative guidance discussions. In addition, it is striking that the 46 patients receiving encouragement and education were ready for discharge an average of 2.7 days before the 51 matched control cases.

Attempts in public health have been made for some years to prepare pregnant women for childbirth and for dealing with expectable problems in the growth and development of their children. Anticipatory guidance techniques are also used in the Peace Corps to prepare volunteers to face the challenges of overseas service. Some of this preparation has been done by psychiatrists in a special mental health sequence in Peace Corps training programs, and a pamphlet, *Adjusting Overseas,*[35] is given to every trainee. It describes the many stresses, such as loneliness, strange living conditions, different value systems, boredom, and lack of obvious signs of accomplishment, which volunteers must expect in their assignments, and tells them that they will probably become depressed, anxious, angry, and confused when exposed to these conditions. The psychiatrist then meets with the trainees in a small group to discuss in advance some of the negative feelings they are likely to have as they go through these difficulties; they may then be better prepared to accept their feelings, to master them, and to seek the emotional support of their associates and of the Peace Corps staff.

CONCEPTS AND EVALUATION

No discussion of primary prevention would be complete without reference to the problems of conceptualization and evaluation, particularly when the focus is on a population. These are the areas where the greatest problems exist and the least work has been done. The conceptual model used in this paper is to divide the environmental influences on human development into long- and short-term factors, and to subdivide the nature of the factors into physical, psychosocial, and sociocultural. Bloom (unpublished), on the other hand, has suggested that one may consider primary prevention programs as focusing on the total community; on individuals who are passing a certain mile-stone in their lives; and on high-risk groups. Bolman and Westman[76] have suggested that preventive programs dealing with young children can be divided into society-centered, family-centered, and child-centered efforts. It is clear that these different conceptualizations are not contradictory, but complementary. The schema used in the present paper focuses attention on the vicissitudes of human growth and development and the forces which foster or impede it, while the other two focus attention on specific goals and methods of programs of primary prevention. Indeed, in the absence of great knowledge as to the etiology of mental illness and psychological maldevelopment, any conceptual framework will be a temporary expedient adopted for pragmatic purposes. As this is the case for all sciences, whether exact and highly developed or primitive and inexact, we should not be too troubled.

The efficacy of preventive efforts has been assessed in too few of the programs discussed in this review. While many ideas about primary prevention seem plausible, are based on clinical judgment, or are transpositions of findings from one area of research to another, we will only gain greater certitude if we make evaluative studies. Yet the problems of evaluation are many, as in evaluating the effects of psychotherapy, but on a much larger scale. This discussion will be brief and focus on the salient issues of goals, controls, and assessment techniques; and the reader is referred to reviews of the field, such as those by Hyman,[77] Freeman,[78] Etzioni,[79] and MacMahon.[80]

The problem of specifying the goals of an intervention program is a particularly knotty one. For example, Brim,[81] in his discussion of parent education, notes that the aims of such education depend not only on the particular psychological theory which one espouses, but also on the values which one holds. It is impossible to educate without advocating, and so too, efforts at prevention involve issues of value. Thus, to express one's grief at a loss may be useful for one's mental health, but it is antithetical to the value of stoicism. Furthermore, the goals of preventive efforts are rarely single and simple; they are usually multiple and complex. As Brim points out, education may influence the parent in the direction of being both more knowledgeable about his influence on his child, and less anxious at the same time. These objectives may in fact conflict; but even if they do not, the results of programs designed to effect them require quite different evaluative techniques. The problems of determining goals thus involves matters of both value orientation and of clarifying the various aims of any given program.

Problems of specifying and obtaining adequate controls are also difficult. Most programs of prevention involve the individual's consent and participation, and it is well known that these are aspects of personality which may influence outcome. If one obtains a person's agreement to participate in a program which will be helpful to him, can one then refuse to let him participate? A choice has to be made whether the control group is to be offered no intervention at all or some placebo program, since there are likely to be effects on individuals from just giving them some attention entirely apart from the specific aims of any given program of prevention. Furthermore, in many programs which last over time, there is the problem of drop-outs. Such individuals clearly do not terminate randomly, and dropping out is likely to be associated with other characteristics of personality which may influence outcome. It is clear that to specify the appropriate controls for use in evaluating attempts at intervention and what program, if any, to offer is difficult, particularly when the focus is on a population.

Bloom (unpublished), who comments that the field is a "nightmare," describes four types of research which often are considered as evaluative: (1) program description; (2) evaluation based on judgments made by recipients; (3) evaluation based on judgments made by professionals; and (4) evaluations based on analysis of objective data without recourse to intervening interpretive judgments. Only the last three can truly be considered evaluative, yet each has its own built-in problems of reliability, validity, and bias. The last type of evaluation, based on objective data, may seem to be the most plausible, yet it too has its problems. For instance, hospitalization rates depend heavily on admission policies; thus, a high rate of admission can lead by a change of administrative policy to many more psychotics living with their families, without affecting the prevalence of psychosis. In this example, it can be seen that seemingly objective data, i.e., admission rates, may be dependent on unseen and unstudied subjective factors of both patients and families, and of professionals. It appears that different methods of evaluation will be most appropriate for different programs—for some, subjective reports by recipients of increased happiness or decreased familial discord will be appropriate; for others, professional assessment of symptom change or increase in IQ; and for still others, lowered rates of suicide. In all cases, it is necessary that evaluation be attempted and focused as far as possible on the specific objectives of the program, so that we may learn which aspect of a given program influences which aspects of its recipients.

In conclusion, in view of the vast amounts of money

being spent on programs which are primarily psychological, social, and rehabilitative in nature, it is useful to consider costs. Sherwood (unpublished data) points out that it is cost per unit of output alone that should be considered. A program which costs little per person and serves large numbers may be highly wasteful if little is accomplished, when compared with a program which spends the same amount of money on far fewer recipients but accomplishes more, not only with each recipient, but in total.

SUMMARY

It is clear from this review of the literature on primary prevention that much has been learned from clinical experience and research; yet, unfortunately, it must be admitted that what is known is often not used. To cite but one example, the short-term effects of hospitalization on infants and small children are well known and thoroughly documented. And yet, it remains true that all too few hospitals take into account the emotional needs of their child patients, and large impersonal institutions exist for the care of the wards of the state. Why this should be so is an important question for psychiatrists to answer. It may well be that we are better prepared and willing to deal with the needs of individual patients than to enter the broad field of implementing social change; yet it is clear that much of the knowledge on primary prevention suggests that we must change institutions, not only individuals. Eisenberg[25] asks, in his presidential address to the American Orthopsychiatric Association, "If not now, when?" Pellagra and cretinism are prevented, not by treating individuals, but by altering the nutritional patterns of groups; so, too, "hospitalism" and the adverse effects of institutionalization can only be prevented by altering organizations. In conclusion, it may be said that while the specific etiological factors which lead to specific mental illnesses are not known and much remains to be learned, a great deal is known about the prevention of psychological maldevelopment, maladaptation, and misery; and much remains undone.

REFERENCES

1. Calhoun, J. B.: "Population Density and Social Pathology," in Duhl, L. J. (ed.): *The Urban Condition,* New York: Basic Books, Inc., 1963, pp. 33-43.

2. Kubzansky, P. E.: "The Effects of Reduced Environmental Stimulation on Human Behavior: A Review," in Biderman, A. D., and Zimmer, H. (eds.): *The Manipulation of Human Behavior,* New York: John Wiley & Sons, Inc., 1961, pp. 51-95.

3. Kleitman, N.: *Sleep and Wakefulness,* ed 2, Chicago: University of Chicago Press, 1965.

4. Hartman, E. L.: The D-State, *New Eng J Med* 273 (2):87-92 (July 8) 1965.

5. Srole, L., et al.: *Mental Health in the Metropolis,* New York: McGraw-Hill Book Company, 1961, vol. 1.

6. Leighton, D., et al.: *The Character of Danger,* New York: Basic Books, Inc., 1963.

7. Moncrieff, A. A.: Treatment of Phenyl Ketonuria: Report to the Medical Research Council of the Conference on Phenyl Ketonuria, *Brit Med J* 1:1691-1697, 1963.

8. Means, J. H., DeGroot, L. J., and Stanbury, J. B.: *The Thyroid and Its Diseases,* ed 3, New York: McGraw-Hill Book Co. Inc., 1963.

9. Wohl, M. D., and Goodhart, R. S. (eds.): *Modern Nutrition and Disease,* Philadelphia: Lea & Febiger, Publishers, 1960.

10. University of Cincinnati: Symposium on Lead, *Arch Environ Health* 8:202-354, 1964.

11. Hess, R. D., and Shipman, V. C.: Early Experience and the Socialization of Cognitive Modes in Children, *Child Res* 36 (4):869-886, 1965.

12. Deutsch, M.: The Role of Social Class in Language Development and Cognition, *Amer J Orthopsychiat* 35:78-87, 1964.

13. John, V. P.: The Intellectual Development of Slum Children: Some Preliminary Findings, *Amer J Orthopsychiat* 33 (5): 813-822 (Oct) 1963.

14. Keller, S.: The Social World of the Urban Slum Child: Some Early Findings, *Amer J Orthopsychiat* 33 (5): 823-831 (Oct) 1963.

15. Weisman, A., and Hackett, T. P.: Psychosis After Eye Surgery: Establishment of a Specific Doctor-Patient Relation in the Prevention and Treatment of "Black Patch Delirium," *New Eng J Med* 258:1284, 1958.

16. Kornfeld, D. S., Zimberg, S., and Malm, J. K.: Psychiatric Complications of Open-Heart Surgery, *New Eng J Med* 273:287-292, 1965.

17. Rice, E. P., and Krakow, S. G.: Hospitalization of a Parent for Mental Illness: A Crisis for Children, read before the 42nd annual meeting of the American Orthopsychiatric Association, New York, March 17-20, 1965.

18. Spitz, R. A.: "Hospitalism: An Inquiry Into the Genesis of Psychiatric Conditions in Early Childhood," in Fenichel, O., et al. (eds); *Psychoanalytic Study of the Child,* New York: International Universities Press, Inc., 1945, vol 1, pp 53-74.

19. Bowlby, E. J. M.: *Maternal Care and Mental Health,* Monograph No. 2, World Health Organization Bulletins, Geneva: World Health Organization, 1951, vol 3, pp 355-533.

20. Provence, S., and Lipton, R. C.: *Infants in Institutions,* New York: International Universities Press, Inc., 1962.

21. Skeels, H. M.: *Adult Status of Children With Contrasting Early Life Experiences: A Follow-Up Study, Monogr Soc Res Child Develop* 31, No. 105, 1966.

22. Wiltse, K. T.: Orthopsychiatric Programs for Socially Deprived Groups, *Amer J Orthopsychiat* 33 (5):806-813 (Oct) 1963.

23. Eisenberg, L.: The Sins of the Fathers: Urban Decay and Social Pathology, *Amer J Orthopsychiat* 32 (1):5-17 (Jan) 1962.

24. Prugh, D., et al.: A Study of Emotional Reactions of Children and Families to Hospitalization and Illness, *Amer J Orthopsychiat* 23:70-106, 1953.

25. Eisenberg, L.: If Not Now, When? *Amer J Orthopsychiat* 32 (5):781-791 (Oct) 1962.

26. Mason, E. A.: The Hospitalized Child—His Emotional Needs, *New Eng J Med* 272(8):406-414 (Feb) 1965.

27. Committee on the College Student: *The College Experience: A Focus for Psychiatric Research* (GAP Report No. 52), New York: Group for the Advancement of Psychiatry, 1962.

28. Committee on the College Student: *Sex and the College Student* (GAP Report No. 60), New York: Group for the Advancement of Psychiatry, 1965.

29. Barger, B.: "The University of Florida Mental Health Program," in *Higher Education and Mental Health,* Gainesville, Fla: University of Florida, 1964.

30. Williams, R. H., Tibbetts, C.; and Donahue, W. (eds.): *The Processes of Aging,* New York: Atherton Press, 1963.

31. French, J. R. P., Jr.: The Industrial Environment and Mental Health, read before the First International Congress of Social Psychiatry, August 1964.

32. Tureen, L., and Wortman, M.: A Program Sponsored by a Labor Union for Treatment and Prevention of Psychiatric Conditions, *Amer J Orthopsychiat* 35 (3):594-597 (April) 1965.

33. Glass, A. J.: "Observations Upon the Epidemiology of Mental Illness in Troops During Warfare," in Walter Reed Army, Institute of Research: *Symposium on Preventive and Social Psychiatry,* Washington: US Government Printing Office, 1958, pp 185-198.

34. Fried, M.: Effects of Social Change on Mental Health, *Amer J Orthopsychiat* 34 (3):3-28, 1964.

35. Caplan, G.: *Principles of Preventive Psychiatry,* New York: Basic Books, Inc., 1964.

36. Lindemann, E.: Symptomatology and Management of Acute Grief, *Amer J Psychiat* 101:141-148, 1944.

37. Engel, G. L.: Is Grief a Disease? *Psychosom Med* 23(1):18-22, 1961.

38. Caplan, G.: Patterns of Parental Response to the Crisis of Premature Birth, Psychiatry 23(4):365-374 (Nov) 1960.

39. Caplan, G., Mason, E. A.; and Kaplan, D. M.: Four Studies of Crisis in Parents of Prematures, *Community Mental Health J* 1(2):149-161 (summer) 1965.

40. Tichener, J. L., and Levine, M.: *Surgery as a Human Experience,* New York: Oxford University Press, 1960.

41. English, J. T., and Colman, J. G.: Biological Adjustment Patterns of Peace Corps Volunteers, *Psychiatric Opinion* 3:29, 1966.

42. Rapoport, R.: Transition From Engagement to Marriage, *Acta Sociol* 8:1-2, 1964.

43. Silber, E., et al.: Adaptive Behavior in Competent Adolescents Coping With the Anticipation of College, *Arch Gen Psychiat* 5:354-365, 1961.

44. Silber, E., et al.: Competent Adolescents Coping With College Decisions, *Arch Gen Psychiat* 5:517-527, 1961.

45. Parad, H. J.: *Crisis Intervention: Selected Readings,* New York: Family Service Association of America, 1965.

46. Rapoport, L.: Working With Families in Crisis: An Exploration in Preventive Intervention, *Social Work* 7:48, 1962.

47. Freud, S.: "Types of Onset of Neurosis" in Strachey, J. (ed and trans): *The Standard Edition of the Complete Psychological Works of Sigmund Freud,* London: Hogarth Press, 1958, vol 12, pp 231-238.

48. Hamburg, D. A.: "Plasma and Urinary Corticosteroid Levels in Naturally Occurring Psychologic Stresses," in Association for Research in Nervous and Mental Disease: *Ultrastructure and Metabolism of the Nervous System,* Baltimore: Williams and Wilkins Company, 1962, vol 40, pp 406-413.

49. Caplan, G.: *An Approach to Community Mental Health,* New York: Grune & Stratton, 1961.

50. Zetzel, E. R.: "Depression and the Incapacity to Bear It," in Schur, M. (ed): *Drives, Affects, Behavior,* New York: International Universities Press, vol 2, 1965.

51. Kiessler, F.: "Is This Psychiatry?" in Goldston, S. E. (ed): *Concepts of Community Psychiatry: A Framework for Training,* Public Health Service Publication No. 1319, Washington: Department of Health, Education and Welfare, 1965, pp 147-157.

52. Faberow, N. L., and Schneidman, E. S.: *The Cry for Help,* New York: McGraw-Hill Book Company, Inc., 1961.

53. Aldrich, C. K.: Homemaker Service: Adjunct in Mental Hygiene and Socio-Psychiatric Rehabilitation, *Progress in Psychotherapy* 4:159-162, 1959.

54. Torric, M. (ed): *The Cruse Club Chronicle: Monthly Newsletter of the Counselling Service for Widows and Their Families,* Richmond, Surrey, England: E. H. Baker & Co. Ltd.

55. Egleson, J., and Egleson, J. F.: *Parents Without Partners,* New York: E. P. Dutton & Company, 1961.

56. Robinson, R., Demarche, D. F., and Wagle, M. K.: *Community Resources in Mental Health,* No. 5, Joint Commission on Mental Illness and Health Monograph Series, New York: Basic Books, Inc., 1960.

57. Klein, D. C., and Lindemann, E.: "Preventive Intervention in Individual and Family Crisis Situations," in Caplan, G. (ed): *Prevention of Mental Disorders in Children,* New York: Basic Books, Inc., 1961.

58. Waldfogel, S., and Gardner, G. E.: "Intervention in Crises as a Method of Primary Prevention," in Caplan, G. (ed): *Prevention of Mental Disorders in Children,* New York: Basic Books, Inc., 1961.

59. Parad, H. J.: The Use of Time-Limited Crisis Intervention in Community Mental Health Programming, *Social Service* Review 40:275-282, 1966.

60. Moore, T.: Difficulties of the Ordinary Child in Adjusting to School, *J Child Psychol Psychiat* 7:17-38, 1966.

61. Bower, E. M.: The Modification, Mediation and Utilization of Stress During the School Years, *Amer J Orthopsychiat* 34(4):667-674 (July) 1964.

62. Bibring, G. L., et al.: "A Study of the Psychological Processes in Pregnancy and of the Earliest Mother-Child Relationship: I. Some Propositions and Comments," in Eissler, R. S., et al. (eds): *Psychoanalytic Study of the Child,* New York: International Universities Press, Inc., 1961, vol 16, pp 9-24.

63. Bibring, G. L., et al.: "A Study of the Psychological Processes in Pregnancy and of the Earliest Mother-Child Relationship: II. Methodological Considerations," in Eissler, R. S., et al. (eds): *Psychoanalytic Study of the Child,* New York: International Universities Press, Inc., 1961, vol 16, pp 25-92.

64. Caplan, G.: *Theory and Practice of Mental Health Consultation,* to be published.

65. Christmas, J. J.: Sociopsychiatric Treatment of the Disadvantaged Psychotic, read before the American Orthopsychiatric Association Meeting, San Francisco, April 13-16, 1966.

66. Pearl, A., and Riessman, F.: *New Careers for the Poor,* New York: The Free Press, 1965.

67. Rieff, R., and Riessman, F.: The Indigenous Non-Professional: A Strategy of Change in Community Action and Community Mental Health Programs, National Institute of Labor Education Report No. 3, Washington, (Nov) 1964.

68. Palmbaum, P. J.: Apprenticeship Revisited, *Arch Gen Psychiat* 13:304-309, 1965.

69. Cadden, V.: "Crisis in the Family" in Caplan, G.: *Principles of Preventive Psychiatry,* New York: Basic Books, Inc., 1964.

70. Ojemann, R. H.: "Investigations on the Effects of Teaching an Understanding and Appreciation of Behavior Dynamics," in Caplan, G. (ed): *Prevention of Mental Disorders in Children,* New York: Basic Books, Inc., 1961, pp 378-397.

71. Morgan, M. I., and Ojemann, R. H.: The Effect of a Learning Program Designed to Assist Youth in an Understanding of Behavior and Its Development, *Child Develop* 13(3):181-194 (Sept) 1942.

72. Biber, B., et al.: *The Psychological Impact of School Experience,* New York: Bank Street College of Education, 1962.

73. Hahn, K.: "Origins of the Outward Bound Trust," in James, D. (ed): *Outward Bound,* London: Routledge & Kegan Paul, 1957.

74. Janis, I. L.: *Psychological Stress,* New York: John Wiley & Sons, 1958.

75. Egbert, L. D., et al.: Reduction of Postoperative Pain by Encouragement and Instruction of Patients, *New Eng J Med* 270:825-827 (April) 1964.

76. Bolman, W. M., and Westman, J. C.: Prevention of Mental Disorder: An Overview of Current Programs, *Amer J Psychiat* 128:1058-1068, 1967.

77. Hyman, E., et al.: *Application of Methods of Evaluation,* Berkeley, Calif: University of California Press, 1965.

78. Freeman, H. E., and Sherwood, C. C.: Research in Large-Scale Intervention Programs, *J Soc Issues* 21:11-28, 1965.

79. Etzioni, A.: Two Approaches to Organizational Analysis: A Critique and a Suggestion, *Admin Sci Quart* 5:257-278 (Sept) 1960.

80. MacMahon, B., Pugh, T. F., and Hutchison, G. B.: Principles in the Evaluation of Community Mental Health Programs, *Amer J Public Health* 7:963-979, 1961.

81. Brim, O. G., Jr.: *Education for Childrearing,* New York: Russell Sage Foundation, 1959.

PRIMARY PREVENTION—MORE COST THAN BENEFIT

Elaine Cumming

A history of primary prevention of mental illness might pass for a thumbnail sketch of the changing value preoccupations of an age. The story moves from the evils of proscribed sex to the virtues of efficiency; from there to the importance of the inner man and finally to the moral value of "the community." If the Victorians did not teach their children that self-control and dutifulness would prevent mental illness, perhaps it was because they did not think in those terms, but the notion of primary prevention had crept in by the time of Bleuler's *fin de siecle* prescription "the avoidance of masturbation, of disappointments in love, of strains or fright are recommendations which can be made with a clear conscience because these are things which should be avoided in all circumstances" (Bleuler, 1950).

By the twenties we were discovering that self-hypnosis, *à la Coué,* for adults and rigorous habit training for children would maintain good mental health. Such optimistic efficiency not surprisingly started to break up during the depression, and by the end of World War II the inner man was paramount and mental health education designed to encourage his expression had taken hold. This stream of. activity, together with a preoccupation with permissiveness in child-raising, characterized the silent, individualistic, in-turned fifties. As approaches to primary prevention, both mental health education and the special emphasis on child-raising, crested during this period and have since receded, so I will refer to them only briefly before going

161

on to what appear to be the two current strategies, crisis intervention and consultation.

I. EARLIER STRATEGIES

Education was the basis of the prevention programs of the recent past, and this education was centered on both child raising and personal practices. Child-raising practices have always been a vehicle for value statements about the good life. It is important to notice, however, that although beliefs about child-raising change, and child-raising practices themselves may change, the rates of mental illness do not appear to change with them (Cumming, 1968). Davis (1965) summarizes the child-raising lore of the 1940's and 1950's as "thermodynamic," being centered on the faith that a warm, loving parent will produce a mentally healthy child, but he also points out that there is little evidence for that faith.*

In the same monograph, Davis reviewed the many attempts to modify personal attitudes and practices through various kinds of exhortations. He concluded that "the important problem, in mental hygiene campaigns concerned with techniques of personal adjustment and prevention of mental illness, is not the appropriate means of communication and persuasion but the fact that mental health educators have nothing concrete and practical to tell the public." Whether or not this little book delivered the *coup de grace* to that kind of mental health education, we will never know, but the tide has certainly ebbed since it appeared. In spite of that, education as a strategy should not be lightly abandoned

* Just in passing, it might be noted that while such an upbringing was explicitly contrasted with the strictness of the earlier behaviorists and the harshness of the Victorians, it was also implicitly contrasted with materialism; "they buy him a roomful of toys but give him no love." Materialism has always been a bugaboo; the Victorians deplored it when they contrasted it with duty and honor, and even the materialistic 20's paid lip service to "the best things in life are free." No matter what has been thought to be the good life, on the surface at least, materialism has been bad. It should also be noted that just as there is no compelling evidence that warmth prevents mental illness there is none that materialism causes it.

just because trivial content has rendered it futile in the past. I will return to this later.

II. NEWER STRATEGIES

The good life has shifted from the self-realization of individuals and is all tied up with the need for community development, community involvement, the redistribution of power (Kaufman, 1969), and saving the world from the violence, corruption, and decay of modern urban life, as well as the fear of a generation that seems actually to be less materialistic than its parents. It is not surprising to find that the prevention of mental illness has draped itself in these more modern garments.

a. Crisis Intervention

We experience the world as in crisis, and it is easy to blame many of our discomforts upon the atmosphere of crisis that is generated by each day's news. Somehow the idea of crisis as an inherent, but undesirable aspect of living has seized us.

The conviction that psychological health is dependent in part upon the successful weathering of life's crises is modern; it seems to have grown from a number of sources, among them ideas of vulnerability at times of change (Lewin, 1951) and ideas of developmental stages (Erickson, 1950). It seems likely from a variety of evidence that rapid treatment of the crisis of acute mental illness is an essential part of the good practice of psychiatry (Cumming and Cumming, 1962; Joint Information Service, 1966), and I explicitly exclude from this discussion consideration of crisis intervention as a therapeutic technique.

Caplan (1964) appears to have given the first impetus to crisis intervention as a *preventive technique among normal people*. It is worth noting, however, before discussing this strategy that most of the changes of status that punctuate an ordinary life span, except perhaps bereavement, would not have been called crises as little as a generation ago. Now, in an age of crises, entering school, puberty, going to college, marriage, parenthood, and retirement all have this label.

A number of descriptions of crisis intervention programs designed to prevent mental illness among normal people who are undergoing such expectable life crises as adolescence, childbirth, marriage, and bereavement can be found in the literature. These programs are lent a certain *prima facie* validity by retrospective clinical reports of psychologically impaired people who have been found not to have resolved such crises. A classical example of this kind of evidence is Lindemann's 1944 report of unresolved grief among bereaved families. Unfortunately, no study was found that had both a baseline measure and evidence that people who did not adequately resolve their grief were later inclined to a variety of psychological disabilities. It is, therefore, not possible to tell whether or not these same people had been psychologically healthy before the bereavement. While useful therapies have been based upon such *post hoc* clinical evidence, it is a doubtful basis indeed for a program of prevention that would in its nature require resources sufficient to serve the enormous populations at risk, very few of whom would be expected to be affected. Even if only "high risk groups" were included, such as widows under 60 years of age, (Silverman, 1967), the ratio of service delivered to illness prevented would be enormous. Similar criticisms of preventive interventions with the parents of premature infants can be made. Although Caplan's group found that they could predict which parents would meet their criteria of good adaptation by examining patterns of "grappling behavior" during the crisis of having a premat re infant (Caplan, 1965), the ability of these people to co₁ ə with this crisis is not, of course, independent of their ge ieral competence before the crisis.* Services routinely supplied to the parents of premature children would be expected to have a very low yield. (Perhaps if obstetricians had more confi-

---

* The psychiatrists' ability to predict simply shows that they are able to discriminate among people of different competencies on the basis of one sampling of behavior, itself no mean feat, but beside the point.

dence in psychiatrists they would refer to them those patients who were not grappling well.) No studies could be found that showed that intervention at the time of normal crisis had any effect upon subsequent mental illness.

There are two further problems to be raised about the use of this kind of intervention as primary prevention in a society in which every individual can expect to pass through a number of changes from one status to another. First, since there are institutional supports for these transitions in a stable society, there does not seem to be any obvious reason why intervention by psychiatrists should be needed, especially since psychiatrists are needed for treating the mentally ill. If society is in such a condition of change that these crises become difficult for a large number of people, a good argument can be made for trying to strengthen the social fabric rather than the population. This is a task that more and more psychiatrists are in fact willing to undertake, and I will return to this new role later than when I discuss consultation. My point here is that primary prevention through crisis intervention is in theory unnecessary in a stable society, and in an unstable one the usefulness of deploying scarce resources for this purpose should have to be demonstrated.

The final objection to crisis intervention as a preventive strategy is perhaps the most important one: in spite of the assumption that in this crisis-ridden world crises are inevitably experienced as strains (Peck, 1968), such evidence as is available about the relationship of stress to psychiatric breakdown suggests that it is not crisis that leads to personality disorganization and psychiatric casualty, but exposure to continued, unremitting stress (Appel and Beebe, 1946; Funkenstein, 1954; Michaux, 1967; Katz, 1970). The literature on this matter might be summed up as, "all that stresses is not strain."

When individuals are under long-continued stress, however, there is an implication of a stressful environment and therefore the implication that psychiatric casualties might be more easily avoided by changing the environment than by strengthening the individual. In a brilliant and influential report on the need for a preventive program in the army, Appel and Beebe (1946) pointed out that only a change in the structure of the environment of infantrymen could reduce psychiatric casualties. In the army, changes in environment can be made by fiat. In civilian life, not only is major change by executive order impossible, but the stresses are more complex.

We take for granted that slums, poverty, deprivation, and humiliation are stresses that are felt as strains whether or not they generate the surplus of mental illness with which they are associated. It is the core of my argument that the urgent moral imperatives of the day arise in revulsion from and fear of the vile conditions in urban slums, and that these morally debasing conditions are therefore assumed to be causing mental illness, just as yesterday strict child-raising practices and repression of hostile impulses were assumed to cause it then.* My guess is that our prevention strategies would be exactly the same even if the statistical associations between slums and rates of schizophrenia were unknown to us. No one knows whether or not vile living conditions actually cause mental illness, but in a civilized society they should be found intolerable just because they are vile. All citizens, not just psychiatrists, should be appalled at them.

If it does turn out to be true that adverse conditions of life cause mental illness, such knowledge will not necessarily help. It is already known that they cause physical illness and mental retardation and are associated with crime, delinquency, despair, suicide, and numbers of other unwanted effects, and always have been. It is clearly not the mandate of any one discipline to remove itself from its central specialty and attend to the moral dilemmas of the nation. We would not be happy if the obstetrician left the ward aide to deliver the

---

* For years the Mental Health Associations of the country distributed "Blondie" comics teaching us how to express our emotions instead of bottling them up.

babies while he was busy organizing the community to fight the conditions that lead to foetal wastage. The world will change but it will be changed by socio-political processes, as it has been in the past. There is a certain arrogance in someone who has been trained to heal the sick imagining that he therefore has an expertise beyond that of any other thoughtful citizen in patching up the cracks in society. Indeed, the naivete of some of the literature in this field must be attributed to this arrogance. When we read that the world can be changed by "altering social arrangements to insure that those who have done the right things are indeed rewarded," and that "a congress on ethics and conduct should be convened to . . . dispel the present confusion about sex and to change society . . ." (Arsenian, 1965), we can only wonder whether members of the psychiatric fraternity and their paraprofessional brothers do not have a trained incapacity to understand the history and the structure of American society.

None of this is prejudicial to the so-called store-front movement. Experiments with new forms are needed. Perhaps psychiatric care ought to be delivered to people close to where they are, and certainly in terms that they can understand and under conditions that do not humiliate and alienate them. Perhaps this means that treatment must sometimes be delivered in the fronts of stores, church basements, and other unorthodox places, and especially that it be given in the evenings and on weekends, but it is my contention that this should be done in the name of giving humane and efficient care to the mentally ill and that pretensions about it preventing mental illness should be abandoned. They should be abandoned not only because the psychiatrist is unlikely to be particularly effective at such preventive tactics but also, and more importantly, because too often in the excitement the patient, especially the chronically ill patient, is forgotten, "merely clinical" activities are discarded, and the psychiatrist is off on one of his moon journeys doctoring society. These journeys are sometimes called consultation.

b. Consultation

The literature on consultation makes depressing reading for anyone interested in evidence. Program descriptions abound, but evaluations of these are lacking, perhaps because it is so difficult to conceive of a method of showing that any mental illness is prevented by consultations of any kind. The reason for this difficulty is that both the method of prevention and the implied etiology of the disease are so diffuse. We seem to have adopted a kind of moral miasma theory of causation (Bloom, 1965) and we are attacking the disease with a general program of uplift. (At one time the word "uplift" must have had the same with-it modernity that "outreach" had a decade ago. They are equally moral terms.) Mental illness is often so mysterious, unpredictable, and threatening to the moral order that until we know more about it, these diffuse moral attitudes may be inevitable.

(i) Case Consultation.   Some of the hundreds of descriptions of consultation programs that fill the journals include interesting typologies, most of which reveal that not all consultation is preventive in intent, and the most interesting of which is four-fold. The first type, case consultation, is an absolutely orthodox component of every branch of medicine and an essential part of good practice. When the target of intervention is someone already impaired, consultation must be considered treatment and not prevention. Even so, there is evidence that agencies can be frustrated by consultation. By the time they call for a consultant they really want to make a referral. Often, they have already used all the techniques of which they are capable, and the psychiatrist cannot add anything to their armamentarium of skills in his consulting capacity. Rabiner (1970) has suggested that psychiatric consultation will be accepted only when direct services are already in effect, and when there is an active demand for the consulting service. Brodsky (1970), in an interesting inter-system analysis, cautions the psychiatrist to respect the roles of other specialists when he

offers his services. In passing, no descriptions of consultation programs being developed in response to a spontaneous community demand could be found. Consultation does not appear to be as good a mousetrap as a treatment program.

(ii) Consultee-oriented   Consultation. "Consultee-oriented" consultation seems to consist of the psychiatrist somehow making the consultee a better and more mature person. Kiyoshi (1969), describing a consultee-oriented consultation says, ". . . when the team meets these people in their offices it adopts an attitude of consultee-oriented consultation rather than patient-oriented consultation. This means that the members of the team will not have any direct contact with the agencies' patients. . . . The consultant is concerned primarily with the growth of the skills of the agency workers and *not with the workers' effectiveness.*"(Italics mine.) Sometimes it is hard to believe that psychiatrists are not actually fleeing from their patients (Kubie, 1971).

Occasionally, somebody describes a consultation program that had unpleasant and unintended consequences, but such authors, though thoughtful and honest, seem never to question the basic utility of their programs. It is difficult, however, for an outsider to know exactly why a psychiatrist is better at improving the skills of a policeman or a school teacher than a school teacher or a policeman is at improving his.

(iii) Educational Consultation.   The third kind of consultation is basically education. The psychiatrist lectures at PTA meetings and any other organizations that invite him in the hope that this will change their practices. As Davis (1965) concluded from his review of the literature, however, "It appears that there is a continuum in degrees of change from beliefs to attitudes to subjective states to practices. Almost all studies of change in information show positive results while . . . studies of change in practice show negative outcomes." Nevertheless, as Davis says, the possession of information is itself valuable because it reassures people

(Nunnally, 1961), sets up realistic standards against which people can measure their own performances, and tends to innoculate against overreaction to stress (Janis, 1958). More research into the long-term effects of specific factual education programs is much needed. The intellect should never be sold too short.

Whether education can ever be specific and rational and still achieve this purpose is perhaps the question. It may be that until we know something more specific about the mental illnesses that remain so hard to control, their implicit threat to society will always evoke moral responses and these will always color educational programs. Perhaps we will never be able to prevent these illnesses until we can cure them.

(iv) Community Consultation.   Finally, in a decade of power to the people (both radicals, and those arch-conservatives, the community establishment), there is community consultation in which the psychiatrist becomes involved in many kinds of groups and organizations for various purposes including that of involving his potential patients in efforts to improve their living conditions (Peck, 1968).

There are three objections to this activity, two of them discussed above. First, it is essentially a reform activity for which a psychiatrist is not trained; second, it distracts him from his core activity which is the care and treatment of the ill. Third, there is no evidence that any of these activities at any time prevented so much as one case of mental illness. Nobody, in fact, appears to be interested in trying to discover the effects of these efforts and it is very doubtful whether such a discovery could be made because a controlled experiment would be almost impossible to arrange.

It is hard to avoid noticing in reviewing the literature that both consultee-oriented and community consultation seem to be models for a pecking order with the psychiatrist at the top. Just as the psychiatrist does not ask the policeman for his advice, so he cannot give his advice to the one group of people who are convinced that their status is higher than his, that is, other practicing medical doctors. As Eisendorfer and Altrocchi (1968) admit, medical doctors should not be included as consultees because they are "ambivalent to the process."

None of this should be taken as a criticism of programs of community development, restoration, and organization, unquestionably good things in their own right, but just as a reflection of the belief that psychiatrists have other things to do and perhaps also that their very presence unnecessarily suppresses the status of people such as social workers, labor organizers, and many others who are better trained for the job.

III. THERE MUST BE A WAY

I have taken a strong position against certain activities undertaken in the name of primary prevention because I think some psychiatrists have lost their way by allowing themselves to become mouthpieces of a popular morality.

In the past we have succeeded in preventing mental illnesses like pellagra, tertiary syphilis, and various toxic conditions, but we have done it in a thoughtful epidemiological way, discriminating between different forms of illness and combining knowledge about distribution with clinical explorations and then working to establish causal linkages between the environment, the individual, and the illness. An excellent summary of successes in primary prevention is given by Eisenberg (1962). Pointing out that psychiatric illnesses are no less psychiatric for having specific etiologies, Eisenberg lists the known successful strategies. These include genetic counseling, protection of the foetus and the neo-nate to avoid neurological damage, and the wider availability of acceptable birth control methods (on the grounds that there is some evidence that unwanted children are particularly liable to emotional disability). Since Eisenberg's review, this strategy has become more important because of evidence that in large families schizophrenics seem to be in the last half of the sibline, (Hinshelwood, 1970), because schizophrenia appears to be familial (Rosenthal, 1968), and because the fertility of schizophrenic women seems to have increased since the development of community care (New Society, 1970). For all our efforts, however, that great foe is still untouched. As Ewalt and Maltsberger (1969) say, ". . . The present state of psychiatric knowledge does not permit the claim that we can prevent the development of schizophrenic illness in any given individual or population." It is in the area of this frustratingly resistant illness that we are most likely to go astray and to invent gratifying methods of prevention because we have no cures.

SUMMARY

1. The effectiveness of popular strategies for the primary preventions of the major mental illnesses has not been tested.

2. These strategies remove needed manpower from the treatment of the mentally ill.

3. The moral and social problems that afflict our society should be attacked because they are insupportable, not because they cause mental illness, which has not been demonstrated.

REFERENCES

Apple, John W., and Gilbert W. Beebe, 1946, Preventive Psychiatry, *Journal of the American Medical Association,* Vol. 131, No. 18, pp. 1469-1475.

Arsenian, John, 1965, Toward Prevention of Mental Illness in the United States, *Community Mental Health Journal,* Vol. 1, No. 4, Winter, pp. 320-325.

Bleuler, E., 1950, *Dementia Praecox.* New York: International Universities Press.

Bloom, Bernard L., 1965, The 'Medical Model,' Miasma Theory, and Community Mental Health, *Community Mental Health Journal,* Vol. 1, No. 4, Winter, pp. 333-338.

Brodsky, Carroll M., 1970, Decision-Making and Role Shifts as They Affect the Consultation Interface, *Archives of General Psychiatry,* Vol. 23, No. 6, December, pp. 559-565.

Caplan, Gerald, Edward A. Mason, and David M. Kaplan, 1965, Four Studies of Crisis in Parents of Prematures, *Community Mental Health Journal,* Vol. 1, No. 2, Summer, pp. 149-161.

Caplan, Gerald, 1964, *Principles of Preventive Psychiatry.* New York: Basic Books.

Cumming, Elaine, 1968, Unsolved Problems of Prevention, *Canada's Mental Health Supplement,* No. 56, January-April.

Cumming, John and Elaine, 1962, *Ego and Milieu.* New York: Atherton.

Davis, James A., 1965, *Education for Positive Mental Health.* Chicago: Aldine.

Eisenberg, Leon, 1962, Preventive Psychiatry, *Annual Review of Medicine,* Vol. 13, pp. 343-360.

Eisendorfer, Carl, John Altrocchi, and Robert F. Young, 1968, Principles of Community Mental Health in a Rural Setting: The Halifax County Program, *Community Mental Health Journal,* Vol. 4, No. 3, June, pp. 211-220.

Erickson, Erik, 1950, *Childhood and Society.* New York: W.W. Norton.

Ewalt, Jack R., and John T. Maltsberger, 1969, "Prevention" in *The Schizophrenic Syndrome,* eds. L. Bellak and L. Loeb. New York: Grune-Stratton. (pp. 757-775).

Funkenstein, Daniel H., Stanley H. King, and Margaret E. Drolette, 1957, *Mastery of Stress.* Cambridge: Harvard University Press.

Hinshelwood, R. D., 1970, The Evidence for a Birth Order Factor in Schizophrenia, *British Journal of Psychiatry,* Vol. 117, No. 538, p. 293.

Janis, I., 1958, *Psychological Stress: Psychoanalytic and Behavioral Studies of Surgical Patients.* New York: John Wiley.

Joint Information Service of the American Psychiatric Association and the National Association for Mental Health, 1966, *The Psychiatric Emergency.* Washington, D. C.

Katz, Jack L., H. Weiner, T. F. Gallagher, and Leon Hellman, 1970, Stress, Distress, and Ego Defenses: Psychoendocrine Response to Impending Breast Tumor Biopsy, *Archives of General Psychiatry,* Vol. 23, No. 2, August, pp. 131-142.

Kaufman, Herbert, 1969, Administrative Decentralization and Political Power, *Public Administration Review,* Vol. XXIX, No. 1, January-February, pp. 3-14.

Kiyoshi, Ogura, and Virgil Bradley, 1967, A Look at the Consultative Process: The Psychiatric Team and Community Agencies, *Psychiatric Quarterly Supplement,* Vol. 41, Part 1, pp. 15-35.

Kubie, L. S., 1971, The Retreat from Patients, *Archives of General Psychiatry,* Vol. 24, No. 2, February, pp. 98-106.

Lewin, Kurt, 1951, *Field Theory in Social Sciences.* New York: Harper.

Lindemann, Erich, 1944, Symptomatology and Management of Acute Grief, *American Journal of Psychiatry,* Vol. 101, pp. 141-148.

Michaux, William W., Kathleen H. Gansereit, Oliver L. McCabe, and Albert Kurland, 1967, The Psychopathology and Measurement of Environmental Stress, *Community Mental Health Journal,* Vol. 3, No. 4, Winter, pp. 358-372.

New Society, 1970, Fertility of the Mentally Ill, January 29th, Vol. 15, No. 383, p. 183.

Nunnally, J. C., Jr., 1961, *Popular Conceptions of Mental Health: Their Development and Change.* New York: Hold, Rhinehart, and Winston.

Peck, Harris B., 1968, The Small Group: Core of the Community Mental Health Center, *Community Mental Health Journal,* Vol. 4, No. 3, June, pp. 191-200.

Rabiner, Charles J., Seymour Silverberg, John W. Galvin, and Leon D. Hankoff, 1970, Consultation or Direct Service, *American Journal of Psychiatry,* Vol. 126, No. 9, March, pp. 1321-1325.

Rosenthal, David, and Seymour S. Kety, 1968, *The Transmission of Schizophrenia.* New York: Pergammon.

Silverman, Phyllis Rolfe, 1967, Services to the Widowed: First Steps in a Program of Preventive Intervention, *Community Mental Health Journal,* Vol. 3, No. 1, Spring, pp. 37-44.

Part V
Extending The Definition Of Mental Health

EXTENDING THE DEFINITION OF MENTAL HEALTH

A limited definition of mental health would confine it to the diagnosis and treatment of traditional diagnostic categories such as neurosis and psychosis. Advocates of extending the definition of mental health indicate that there are virtually no limits as to the areas in which there are important mental health implications. Social organizations, racial discrimination, violence, and education are a few of the areas to which mental health practitioners might apply their expertise and contribute to an understanding and solution of problems. Advocates feel that the social problems of our society are so pressing that the mental health practitioner can no longer confine himself only to diagnosing and treating patients.

Opponents attack an extended definition of mental health from a variety of fronts. On one side there are those who believe that mental health workers do not belong in fields in which they have no specialized knowledge or skills. The community organizer, criminologist, civil rights leader, educator, and politician are examples of those who are far more knowledgeable and adept in their own areas than the mental health worker, who, when he goes into their fields, is acting presumptuously. Also, the mental health worker is likely to stress individual psychopathology when the more important aspects of the situation may be variables such as power politics, economics, urban decay, and institutional rigidity.

Others attack an extended definition of mental health on the grounds that it is likely to give rise to mental health practitioners in social control roles. Mental health practitioners traditionally serve their clients in a mutually agreed-upon, circumscribed manner with ethical standards governing the conditions and nature of the relationship. When mental health practitioners become involved in other areas in which their activity may result in political, economic, educational, etc., decisions affecting the lives of people and these activities and decisions are not subject to the usual professional limitations and ethical standards then, in effect, mental health practitioners are controlling people without their consent, may be infringing on people's civil rights, and doing so under the banner of vague and unproven mental health principles.

Dr. Bertram S. Brown, Director, National Institute of Mental Health, is a well-known advocate of mental health as a force that can humanize the social changes and upheavals of our times. At numerous conferences covering topics as far-ranging as criminal justice, pesticides, discrimination against minority groups, and space exploration, Dr. Brown has pointed out the mental health implications. In the article that follows, Dr. Brown demonstrates how broad he believes the boundaries of mental health to be.

Possibly the best known challenger of the assumptions made about "mental health" and "illness" is Dr. Thomas S. Szasz, Professor of Psychiatry, Upstate University of New York in Syracuse. He has vigorously fought for patients' rights and against what he sees as the encroachments of psychiatry on civil liberties. In "The Mental Health Ethic," Dr. Szasz warns that community psychiatry has become largely a means of controlling the individual for socio-economic and political ends.

EXTENDING THE DEFINITION OF MENTAL HEALTH

Bertram S. Brown

The issue of the definition of mental health is a basic one, with the variation ranging from the extreme of the quality of life, or the ecosystem of the universe, to the illness or disturbed behavior of an individual and the psychological and biological correlates of the individual within that range. In individual illness and the ecosphere we have the organizations that have mental health as a common concern. For example, we might have a mental health center that specializes in treatment of mentally ill people, depressed psychotics or neurotics, or we might have a National Institute of Mental Health which spends considerable time looking into the relevant aspects of the Alaskan pipeline, the ecosphere, the relationship of Indians, turfs, and tundra. The evolution of this definition of mental health so that it extends to what we now call environmental concerns of the quality of life is long-standing and based on the fact that the concerns of the human being range this far. Looked upon from a broad point of view, the definition of mental health will of necessity involve itself in other social systems. If one truly is to affect the quality of life, one must have an effect on institutions which themselves are prime movers of the determinants of quality of life.

As I stated in a recent address,[1] organizations as well as individuals have felt the impact of rapid social change. Each organization thinks it is going through its own unique crisis. The alphabet soup of the APA, the ASA, the AMA, and others do have certain similarities in their organizational crises. Each of the organizations has within it a militant social action group that feels that the time for justice, for equality, for decency, for deep concern for black Americans and other minority groups has come and *now*. Either the parent body must recognize they are right or they threaten to splinter or leave the organization.

On the other extreme are the methodologists, the ritualists who feel that no change is needed or possible and that it is certainly not within the purview of the professional role. They grant the right of concern to citizens and humans, but never confuse the issue by considering the possibility that the professional is simultaneously a citizen and a human being. And, in the middle, is the large band of apathetic practitioners who are passive rather than active.

Each of the organizations realizes that something must be done. Drop-outs must be brought back in; youth must want to come in. The solution for some has been to retreat, not from the issues, but to a place where top leadership gathers to hammer out real organizational changes. I have dealt at length elsewhere with what I call the "organization and reorganization crisis." I have briefly used the schools and professional organizations only as examples. Governmental agencies—State, local, and Federal—corporations, businesses, all organizations are undergoing these difficult shifts in keeping with the demands of our age. From a national perspective it is clear that fundamental changes are taking place in our most basic structures—in the relationship of executive, legislative, and judicial branches and between the Federal government, the States, and the cities.

Briefly summarized, the struggle between mental illness and mental health on a public health scale may be seen as involving two major campaigns. One might be likened to an air battle; it is a conceptual struggle over differences in approach to social problems. The other is more like traditional ground warfare. In this, the mental health agency represents only one of the many interest groups in the struggle for power and authority. Inasmuch as all have ethical goals—to benefit the sick, the aging, the alcoholic, the addict, the delinquent, the retarded—the various groups may well discover ways to cooperate to help people who are, after all, the object of their common concern.

But even under optimal conditions, autonomy will remain a source of disagreement. Since each group is concerned with its hierarchical position and jurisdictional power, the battles remain surprisingly intense and chronic. Accordingly, these struggles must be taken into account by those concerned with the development of comprehensive mental health programs. In addition, issues of administrative leadership and control play a significant role in molding the work environment of practicing clinicians.

The issue is: who is to help make decisions when the authorities disagree or become lost in organizational warfare? In our country the answer is clear—the citizen consumer and his representatives.

These issues and changes—the same ferment and discord and the same radical crises—are taking place in our universities. They are taking place in governments at the State and local level. They are taking place in professional organizations, and they are taking place in many citizen organizations as they renew themselves and reorganize to meet the tremendous tasks of the latter third of the twentieth century.

To meet this challenge, mental health organizations and associations across the land can and must share in resolving some of the great questions raised by the twentieth century: how to effect broad social purposes without forgetting the individual; how to work together for broad goals that will affect and improve individual lives; how to use limited resources effectively; how to be hard-nosed but not hard-hearted.

One target in mental health is the dark side of man's moon; our goal is to alleviate human misery and suffering. Yet we recognize that our concern must encompass the entire globe—the dark side and the light side. It must encompass not only mental illness but mental health as well; not only treatment but prevention; not only prevention in the young, but rehabilitation in the old.

The most critical dimension to the success of mental

health programs is comprehensive, total caring. We all must care. To professionals and patients alike, questions of serving or of being served, all depend to a great degree on that large and at times invisible force: citizen support and action.

Concomitant with the expansion of treatment services in this country, equal effort must be given to development of preventive measures. Mental health professional and citizen alike must intervene in those situations which we know pose serious adjustment problems. Frustration, loneliness, insecurity, impersonalization, tension, and lack of job or success at school—all are associated with personal adjustment. In our present society we can identify areas which impinge on this personal adjustment. Shifting populations, new communities arising overnight, crowded urban areas, materialistic demands on the family, vastly changing job satisfaction, expanding school populations (leading to the fear of loss of individuality), international tensions, academic competition, accelerated living pace, the apparently disappearing 'good neighbor'—all present situations which can cause the breakdown of the individual. What special role of early intervention, of human support, of preventive guidance can citizen groups offer? What special meaning does the organization have for the individual member? Is there a need for extending the organization's helpful hand to the nonjoiner?

The 1970 President's Task Force on the Mentally Handicapped,[2] in which I served as Executive Secretary, was acutely aware of the close relationship between social problems and mental disability. Some of the major social problems and their mental health implications as stated by the President's Task Force and its recommendations follow:

> The reciprocal relationship between mental disability and social problems such as racism, poverty, violence, crime and delinquency, and overcrowding is real and complex. Racism is declared by many authorities to be the Nation's number one mental health problem. Substandard housing and education, which are the correlates of racism and poverty, are associated with higher rates of mental retardation and mental illness. Violence, ranging from

civil disorders to street crimes, from wars to assassinations, causes mental anguish. Mental instability, in certain cases, causes violence. Environmental pollution has its effects on both body and mind. Individuals impaired—physically, mentally, or emotionally—by environmental and social outrages cannot function efficiently as citizens to correct them.

It is inappropriate to rest the case for improving social conditions solely on the rationale of preventing mental retardation and mental illness. Yet improvement of these conditions will help substantially to prevent mental disability. Conversely, programs directed towards preventing mental retardation and mental illness will improve social conditions.

Poverty

The mechanisms by which poverty contributes to mental disability are subtle at times, as in the effect of malnutrition on brain and intellectual development, and clear at other times, as when poor housing and inadequate child rearing lead to ingestion of lead paint chips, causing bone and brain damage. Other sequelae of poverty are less obviously biological in their operations, but as profound in their impact. There is evidence that the majority of persons with minor forms of mental retardation come from poverty areas. Further, children raised in an atmosphere of hopelessness and apathy, or in chronic anxiety and surrounding hostility, do not easily develop into mature, stable citizens. And children whose lives, through poverty, are dominated by the need for day-to-day survival are unlikely to acquire a concern for others and a respect for law and order.

Poverty is the most important single factor in the production of the social ills.

Violence

National concern over tragic individual and collective acts of violence led to the Kerner and Eisenhower Commissions. Their reports stress underlying causes of violence, including alienation, lack of nonviolent options for certain oppressed groups, increasing polarization of racial attitudes and, therefore, increasing fear, and growing distrust of some governmental institutions.

Continued Presidential leadership is recommended in a national campaign to understand and reduce domestic violence through biological and social research; violence prevention centers, ombudsmen and other such innovative aids to protect the dignity and prevent further alienation of oppressed groups; effective gun controls, and general attention to reducing the rhetoric of violence and the portrayal of violence as a method of problem-solving in America.

Racism

Although opportunities for adequate housing, education, and jobs have improved for minority people in the last decade, true equal opportunity remains a goal to be reached.

The obviously degrading, humiliating discrepancy in opportunity is a serious frustration to the dignity and mental health of all citizens. The effect on children of minority groups is even more profound and tragic. The shortsighted, irrational, prejudicial attitudes of many Americans, attitudes which too often have been nurtured by the family, church and school, seriously interfere with our maturing into a nation of humane, healthy individuals.

Antisocial Behavior

Delinquent and criminal behavior is usually viewed as the end result of interactions among a host of factors—biological, psychological, social, cultural. While the exact nature of these interactions is poorly understood, there is general agreement that behaviors violating socio-legal norms are often symptomatic—as mental illness often is—of social as well as individual distress and dysfunction. These are deviant behaviors. Whether or not they are also labeled delinquent or criminal behaviors can depend in some cases on what jurisdiction or agency is doing the labeling. In any event, they have rightly been the concern of our mental health system. With knowledge of the roots of problem behavior increasing, and with the police and the courts looking more and more frequently to mental health agencies for assistance, this concern is on the rise.

The Nation's mental health system should have the means to inquire much more fully into the causes of anti-social behavior, the most effective ways of preventing it, and the most fruitful policies and techniques for rehabilitating those who have engaged in it. And the juvenile and criminal justice systems should apply much more extensively what is already known about these problems, particularly the rehabilitation of young delinquents and pre-delinquents. The mental health system and the juvenile and criminal justice systems should continue and further improve efforts to work much more closely together on problems of mutual concern.

Recent research suggests that, for those able to use such services, increasing emphasis should be placed on intensive, community-based treatment programs. These can rehabilitate more people at less cost. Equally important, such programs prevent exposure to the atmosphere of penal institutions, which too often foster emotional disorders and criminality.

Research points also to ways of making programs in prisons and reformatories more effective. A pilot project of

self-instruction and vocational training in one State correc-
tional center, for example, led not only to a substantial
increase in earnings when the offenders were released but
also to a substantial decrease in the recidivism rate.
Efforts to tailor the treatment to the type of individual
seem another promising approach.

   While acknowledging the needs of the criminal justice
system in coping with the problem of crime, at the same
time, increased emphasis should be given to crime and
delinquency as a mental health problem.

In addition to the social problems mentioned by the
Presidential Task Force, other examples come readily to
mind.

An example of moving into other social systems that
have implications for mental health is the area of alcoholism, where very specifically the problem of the drunk
driver and traffic safety are closely related. Here we find
that both the resources and the responsibility (legal and
otherwise) rest on the Departments of Transportation
(state, local,and federal), which are engaged in activities
having mental health aspects, such as kinds of tests,
training of safety officers, the writing of law, and sets of
legal behavioral issues. Thus this would be another
example of the expanding boundaries of mental health.

From this point of view one can easily give examples of
aspects of education, housing, law, and violence; there is
no limit in essence to the mental health implications of
other social activities. There are areas here that have not
been explored as yet in any significant way, but which
would yield much to creative efforts. I recall, for example,
dealing with a man who focused on the fact that there
are several hundred thousand bankruptcy petitions filed.
On looking at bankruptcy as a high-risk, high-vulnera-
bility mental health incident, one might find a very rich
way of having impact on the mental health of
populations by moving into the banking and finance
field. And yet, at this point I know of no organized approach towards loan companies in the whole field of
loans and finance. We readily could examine the role of
the small town bank or bankers as mental health agents.
I see no literature on the bankers, yet we find that in
small communities the person who is analogous to the

practitioner or the clergyman is the banker who deals with new business ventures, divorce, bankruptcy, and other important matters. I know of no consultation program available to the banker. So here we have another potential major routing of mental health knowledge into finance, money, and banking. It further reinforces my belief that mental health boundaries ought to be expanded.

The basic thesis of this point of view in mental health is that there is no area of human endeavor which does not have meaningful mental health implications. Take, for example, mental health implications of veterinary practice. It is well known in veterinary practice that there are several "syndromes." We have the pre-child pet of the young married couple, where the pet is in essence a "practice child." We have the "empty nest" pet owner, where a family has brought up children who have left the house and the parents take a pet for the first time. We have the middle-aged or late middle-aged couple having a pet offering special care problems. We have the pet owners who are single men and single women; their taking a pet has certain implications—psychodynamic and otherwise. Research is still to be done to determine the different characteristics of pet owners who favor one kind of animal, such as birds-versus-cats-versus-turtles. We then could turn to the veterinary aspects of horses and cows and large animals or whatever, or of the mental health aspects of veterinarians themselves who chose to work with different species and different animals. One could go on at length and look at the interaction of man and animal as an extension of the human condition, or even taking into the ecological framework the dependence of species. Thus the mental health aspects of veterinary medicine are clear-cut and important. But as far as I am aware they are unexplored.

Another situation which attracted international attention in terms of mental health aspects of man's new endeavors occurred in the events that resulted in a consideration of sex in the space program. Originally in 1967, I was asked to consult on a planned five-man spaceship flight to Mars. The issue at that time was how to

Extending the Definition of Mental Health   187

mix the skills of astronaut, pilot, physiologist, and others so that if any one person became sick or ill, the skills of the other four would overlap those of the fifth. The round trip to Mars was to take roughly nine months and thus involved the problems of small group dynamics, living in a small space, and others that have now become familiar since the moon flights. I added the question of what would be the impact of bringing a woman along on the trip to Mars. And then I did an exploration as to whether it ought to be one woman, two women, or three women, or possibly a man and/or woman, and if so, what age. This eventually brought the problem down to the small group dynamic, the change of tone, people living in small space, but also into some subsidiary issues such as the question of whether orgasm in the weightless state or under other conditions was more pleasurable. We then began to look into the future and see the possibilities of having space platforms where people who were severely handicapped with angina would be capable of carrying out the sexual act. This is given as a serious but perhaps humorous example of some of the mental health implications of the space program.

I have attempted to go beyond prevention and look creatively at promoting mental health. There are dangers of professional heresy in this approach but the risk is worth it. The gravity of the problems facing us requires that we go beyond limited, conventional boundaries.

REFERENCES

1. Brown, Bertram S., *Mental Health and Social Change,* Reprinted by the U.S. Department of Health, Education and Welfare with the permission of the Hogg Foundation of Mental Health, U.S. Government Printing Office, Washington, D.C., 1970.

2. *Action Against Mental Disability, The Report of The President's Task Force on the Mentally Handicapped,* U.S. Government Printing Office, Washington, D.C., September 1970.

THE MENTAL HEALTH ETHIC*

Thomas S. Szasz

Let us begin with some definitions. *Webster's Third New International Dictionary* (unabridged), ethics is "the discipline dealing with what is good and bad or right and wrong or with moral duty and obligation . . ."; it is also "a group of moral principles or set of values . . ." and "the principles of conduct governing an individual or a profession: standards of behavior. . . ."

Ethics is thus a distinctly human affair. There are "principles of conduct" governing individuals and groups, but there are no such principles governing the behavior of animals, machines, or stars. Indeed, the word "conduct" implies this: only persons *conduct* themselves; animals *behave,* machines *function,* and stars *move.*

Is it too much to say, then, that any human behavior that constitutes conduct—which, in other words, is a product of choice or potential choice, and not simply of a reflex—is, *ipso facto,* moral conduct? In all such conduct, considerations of good and bad, or right and wrong, play a role. Logically, its study belongs in the domain of ethics. The ethicist is a behavioral scientist par excellence.

If we examine the definition and practice of psychiatry, however, we find that in many ways it is a covert redefinition of the nature and scope of ethics. According to Webster's, psychiatry is "a branch of medicine that deals with the science and practice of treating mental,

* Reprinted from *Ideology and Insanity,* Chapter 3, with permission of author and publisher, Doubleday & Company, Inc., Garden City, New York, 1970.

emotional, or behavioral disorders esp. as originating in endogenous causes or resulting from faulty interpersonal relationships"; further, it is "a treatise or text on or theory of the etiology, recognition, treatment, or prevention of mental, emotional, or behavioral disorder or the application of psychiatric principles to any area of human activity (social psychiatry)"; thirdly, it is "the psychiatric service in a general hospital (this patient should be referred to psychiatry)."

The nominal aim of psychiatry is the study and treatment of mental disorders. But what are mental disorders? To accept the existence of a class of phenomena called "mental diseases," rather than to inquire into the conditions under which some persons may designate others as "mentally ill," is the decisive step in the embracing of the mental health ethic.[1] If we take the dictionary definition of this discipline seriously, the study of a large part of human behavior is subtly transferred from ethics to psychiatry. For while the ethicist is supposedly concerned only with normal (moral) behavior, and the psychiatrist only with abnormal (emotionally disordered) behavior, the very distinction between the two rests on ethical grounds. In other words, the assertion that a person is mentally ill involves rendering a moral judgment about him. Moreover, because of the social consequences of such a judgment, both the "mental patient" and those who treat him as one become actors in a morality play, albeit one written in a medical-psychiatric jargon.

Having removed mentally disordered behavior from the purview of the ethicist, the psychiatrist has had to justify his reclassification. He has done so by redefining the quality or nature of the behavior he studies: whereas the ethicist studies moral behavior, the psychiatrist studies biological or mechanical behavior. In Webster's words, the psychiatrist's concern is with behavior "originating in endogenous causes or resulting from faulty interpersonal relationships." We should fasten our attention here on the words "causes" and "resulting." With these words, the transition from ethics to physiology, and hence to medicine and psychiatry, is securely completed.

Ethics is meaningful only in a context of self-governing individuals or groups exercising more or less free, uncoerced choices. Conduct resulting from such choices is said to have reasons and meanings, but no causes. This is the well-known polarity between determinism and voluntarism, causality and free will, natural science and moral science.

Defining psychiatry in the above way leads not only to a reapportionment of disciplines taught in universities, but also promotes a point of view about the nature of some types of human behavior, and about man in general.

By assigning "endogenous causes" to human behavior, such behavior is classified as *happening* rather than as *action*. Diabetes mellitus is a disease caused by an endogenous lack of enzymes necessary to metabolize carbohydrates. In this frame of reference, the endogenous cause of a depression must be either a metabolic defect (that is, an antecedent chemical event) or a defect in "interpersonal relationships" (that is, an antecedent historical event). Future events or expectations are excluded as possible "causes" of a feeling of depression. But is this reasonable? Consider the millionaire who finds himself financially ruined because of business reverses. How shall we explain his "depression" (if we so want to label his feeling of dejection)? By regarding it as the result of the events mentioned, and perhaps of others in his childhood? Or as the expression of his view of himself and of his powers in the world, present and future? To choose the former is to redefine ethical conduct as psychiatric malady.

The healing arts—especially medicine, religion, and psychiatry—operate within society, not outside it. Indeed, they are an important part of society. It is not surprising, therefore, that these institutions reflect and promote the primary moral values of the community. Moreover, today, as in the past, one or another of these institutions is used to mold society by supporting certain values and opposing others. What is the role of psychiatry in promoting a covert system of ethics in contemporary American society? What are the moral values it espouses and imposes on society? I shall try to suggest

some answers by examining the position of certain representative psychiatric works and by making explicit the
nature of the mental health ethic. And I shall try to show
that in the dialogue between the two major ideologies of
our day—individualism and collectivism—the mental
health ethic comes down squarely on the side of
collectivism.

II

Men desire freedom and fear it. Karl R. Popper speaks
of the "enemies of the open society,"[2] and Erich Fromm
of those who "escape from freedom."[3] Craving liberty
and self-determination, men desire to stand alone as individuals, but, fearing loneliness and responsibility, they
wish also to unite with their fellow men as members of a
group.

Theoretically, individualism and collectivism are
antagonistic principles: for the former, the supreme
values are personal autonomy and individual liberty, for
the latter, solidarity with the group and collective
security. Practically, the antagonism is only partial:
man needs to be both—alone, as a solitary individual,
and with his fellow man as a member of a group.
Thoreau at Walden Pond and the man in the gray
flannel suit in his bureaucratic organization are two
ends of a spectrum: most men seek to steer a course
between these extremes. Individualism and collectivism
may thus be pictured as the two shores of a fast-moving
river, between which we—as moral men—must navigate.
The careful, the timid, and perhaps the "wise" will take
the middle course: like the practical politician, such a
person will seek accommodation to "social reality" by
affirming and denying both individualism and collectivism.

Although, in general, an ethical system that values individualism will be hostile to one that values
collectivism, and vice versa, an important difference
between the two must be noted: In an individualistic
society, men are not prevented by force from forming
voluntary associations, nor are they punished for

assuming submissive roles in groups. In contrast, in a collectivistic society, men are forced to participate in certain organizational activities, and are punished for pursuing a solitary and independent existence. The reason for this difference is simple: as a social ethic, individualism seeks to minimize coercion and fosters the development of a pluralistic society; whereas collectivism regards coercion as a necessary means for achieving desired ends and fosters the development of a singularistic society.

The collectivist ethic is exemplified in the Soviet Union, as in the case of Iosif Brodsky. A twenty-four-year-old Jewish poet, Brodsky was brought to trial in Leningrad for "pursuing a parasitic way of life." The charge stems from "a Soviet legal concept that was enacted into law in 1961 to permit the exiling of city residents not performing 'socially useful labor.' "[4]

Brodsky had two hearings, the first on February 18 and the second on March 13, 1964. The transcript of the trial was smuggled out of Russia and its translation published in *The New Leader*.[5] In the first hearing Brodsky was vaguely accused of being a poet and of not doing more "productive" work. At its conclusion, the judge ordered Brodsky to be sent "for an official psychiatric examination during which it will be determined whether Brodsky is suffering from some sort of psychological illness or not and whether this illness will prevent Brodsky from being sent to a distant locality for forced labor. Taking into consideration that from the history of his illness it is apparent that Brodsky has evaded hospitalization, it is hereby ordered that division No. 18 of the militia be in charge of bringing him to the official psychiatric examination."[6]

This point of view is characteristic of the collectivist ethic. It is also indistinguishable from that of contemporary American institutional psychiatry. In both systems, a person who has harmed no one but is considered "deviant" is defined as mentally ill; he is ordered to submit to psychiatric examination; if he resists, this is viewed as a further sign of his mental abnormality.[7]

Brodsky was found guilty and sent "to a distant locality for a period of five years of enforced labor."[8] His sentence, it should be noted, was at once therapeutic, in that it sought to promote Brodsky's "personal well-being," and penal, in that it sought to punish him for the harm he had inflicted on the community. This, too, is the classic collectivist thesis: what is good for the community is good for the individual. Since the individual is denied any existence apart from the group, this equation of the one with the many is quite logical.

Another Russian man of letters, Valeriy Tarsis, who had published a book in England describing the predicament of writers and intellectuals under the Khrushchev regime, was incarcerated in a mental hospital in Moscow. It may be recalled that the American poet Ezra Pound had been dealt with in the same way: he was incarcerated in a mental hospital in Washington, D.C.[9] In his autobiographical novel, *Ward 7,* Tarsis gives the impression that involuntary mental hospitalization is a widely used Soviet technique for repressing social deviance.[10]

It seems clear that the enemy of the Soviet state is not the capitalist entrepreneur, but the lonely worker—not the Rockefellers, but the Thoreaus. In the religion of collectivism, heresy is individualism: the outcast par excellence is the person who refuses to be a member of the team.

I shall argue that the main thrust of contemporary American psychiatry—as exemplified by so-called community psychiatry—is toward the creation of a collectivist society, with all this implies for economic policy, personal liberty, and social conformit .

III

If by "community psychiatry" we mean mental health care provided by the community through public funds—rather than by the individual or by voluntary groups through private funds—then community psychiatry is as old as American psychiatry. (In most other countries, too, psychiatry began as a community enterprise and never ceased to function in that role.)

Fresh as the term "community psychiatry" is, many psychiatrists freely admit that it is just another slogan in the profession's unremitting campaign to sell itself to the public. At the fourth annual meeting of the Association of Medical Superintendents of Mental Hospitals, the main topic was community psychiatry—"What it is and what it isn't."[11]

"What is community psychiatry?" asked the director of an eastern state hospital. His answer: "I went to two European congresses this summer and I don't know what is meant by the term. . . . When people talk about it, it is rarely clear what it is."[12] To a psychiatrist in a midwestern state, "Community psychiatry . . . means that we collaborate within the framework of existing medical and psychiatric facilities."[13] This view was supported by a psychiatrist from an eastern state hospital who asserted, "In Pennsylvania, the state hospitals are already serving the communities in which they are located. . . . They have been carrying out community psychiatry."[14] Such is the path of progress in psychiatry.

What I found particularly disturbing in this report was that, although many who attended the meeting were uncertain about what community psychiatry is or might be, all declared their firm intention to play a leading role in it. Said a psychiatrist from a midwestern state hospital: "What community psychiatry is, whatever it becomes, we'd better have a part in it. We'd better assume leadership or we will get the part relegated to us. We should be functioning as community mental hospitals. If we sit back and say we are not community mental health centers, we will have a great many people telling us what to do."[15] The president of the medical superintendents' organization then called upon the members to "assume a role of leadership." There was general agreement on this: "Unless we participate and take a dominant part, we will be relegated to the bottom of the heap,"[16] warned a psychiatrist from a midwestern state hospital.

If this is community psychiatry, what is new about it? Why is it praised and recommended as if it were some novel medical advance that promises to revolutionize the "treatment" of the "mentally ill"? To answer these questions would require an historical study of our subject, which I shall not attempt here.[17] Let it suffice to note the specific forces that launched community psychiatry as a discrete movement or discipline. These forces are of two kinds—one political, the other psychiatric.

The social policies of modern interventionist liberalism, launched by Franklin D. Roosevelt in this country, received powerful reinforcement during the presidency of John F. Kennedy. President Kennedy's Message to Congress on "Mental Illness and Mental Retardation" on February 5, 1963, reflects this spirit. Although the care of the hospitalized mentally ill has been traditionally a welfare-state operation—carried out through the facilities of the various state departments of mental hygiene and the Veterans Administration—he advocated an even broader program, supported by public funds. Said the President: "I propose a national mental health program to assist in the inauguration of a wholly new emphasis and approach to care for the mentally ill. ... Government at every level—federal, state, and local—private foundations and individual citizens must face up to their responsibilities in this area."[18]

Gerald Caplan, whose book Robert Felix called the "Bible ... of the community mental health worker," hailed this message as "the first official pronouncement on this topic by the head of a government in this or any other country."[19] Henceforward, he added, "the prevention, treatment, and rehabilitation of the mentally ill and the mentally retarded are to be considered a community responsibility and not a private problem to be dealt with by individuals and their families in consultation with their medical advisers."[20]

Without clearly defining what community psychiatry is, or what it can or will do, the enterprise is proclaimed good merely because it is a team effort, involving the community and the government, and not a personal effort, involving individuals and their voluntary associations. We are told that the promotion of "community mental health" is so complex a problem that it requires the intervention of the government—but that the individual citizen is responsible for its success.

Community psychiatry is barely off the drawing boards; its nature and achievements are but high-flown phrases and utopian promises. Indeed, perhaps the only thing clear about it is its hostility to the psychiatrist in private practice who ministers to the individual patient: he is depicted as one engaged in a nefarious activity. His role has more than a slight similarity to that of Brodsky, the parasite-poet of Leningrad. Michael Gorman, for example, quotes approvingly Henry Brosin's reflections about the social role of the psychiatrist: "There is no question that the challenge of the role of psychiatry is with us all the time. The interesting thing is what we will be like in the future. Not the stereotypes and strawmen of the old AMA private entrepreneurs."[21]

I have cited the views of some of the propagandists of community psychiatry. But what about the work itself? Its main goal seems to be the dissemination of a collectivistic mental health ethic as a kind of secular religion. I shall support this view by quotations from the leading textbook of community psychiatry, *Principles of Preventive Psychiatry,* by Gerald Caplan.

What Caplan describes is a system of bureaucratic psychiatry in which more and more psychiatrists do less and less actual work with so-called patients. The community psychiatrist's principal role is to be a "mental health consultant"; this means that he talks to people, who talk to other people, and finally someone talks to, or has some sort of contact with, someone who is considered actually or potentially "mentally ill." This scheme works in conformity with Parkinson's Law:[22] the expert at the top of the pyramid is so important and so busy that he needs a huge army of subordinates to help him, and his subordinates need a huge army of second-order subordinates, and so on. In a society faced with large-scale unemployment due to automation and great technological advances, the prospect of a "preventive" mental health industry, ready and able to absorb a vast amount of manpower, should be politically attractive indeed. It is. Let us now look more closely at the actual work of the community psychiatrist.

According to Caplan, a main task of the community psychiatrist is to provide more and better "sociocultural supplies" to people. It is not clear what these supplies are. For example, "the mental health specialist" is described as someone who "offers consultation to legislators and administrators and collaborates with other citizens in influencing governmental agencies to change laws and regulations."[23] In plain English, a lobbyist for the mental health bureaucracy.

The community psychiatrist also helps "the legislators and welfare authorities improve the moral atmosphere in the homes where [illegitimate] children are being brought up and to influence their mothers to marry and provide them with stable fathers."[24] Although Caplan mentions the community psychiatrist's concern with the effects of divorce upon children, there is no comment about advising women who want help in securing divorces, abortions, or contraceptives.

Another function of the mental health specialist is to review "the conditions of life of his target group in the population and then influence[s] those who help to determine these conditions so that their laws, regulations, and policies . . . are modified in an appropriate direction."[25] Caplan emphasizes that he is not advocating government by psychiatrists; he is aware that the psychiatrist may thus become the agent or spokesman of certain political or social groups. He disposes of the problem by declaring that every psychiatrist must make this decision for himself, and that his book is not addressed to those who wish to provide services for special-interest groups, but rather to "those who direct their efforts primarily to the reduction of mental disorder in our communities."[26] But he admits that the distinction between psychiatrists who exploit their professional knowledge in the service of an organization and "those who work in the organization in order to achieve the goals of their profession" is not that simple in practice. For example, commenting on the role of consulting psychiatrists in the Peace Corps, he blandly observes that their success "is not unassociated with the fact that they were able to wholeheartedly accept the major goals of that organization, and their enthusiasm was quickly perceived by its leaders."[27]

On the psychiatrist's proper role in the medical clinics of his community (specifically in relation to his function in a well-baby clinic, seeing a mother who has a "disturbed" relationship with her child), Caplan writes: "If the preventive psychiatrist can convince the medical authorities in the clinics that his operations are a logical extension of traditional medical practice, his role will be sanctioned by all concerned, including himself. All that remains for him to do is to work out the technical details."[28]

But this is precisely what I regard as the central question: Is so-called mental health work "a logical extension of traditional medical practice," either preventive or curative? I say it is not a logical but a rhetorical extension of it.[29] In other words, the practice of mental health education and community psychiatry is not medical practice, but moral suasion and political coercion.

IV

As was pointed out earlier, mental health and illness are but new words for describing moral values. More generally, the semantics of the mental health movement is but a new vocabulary for promoting a particular kind of secular ethic.

This view may be supported in several ways. Here I shall try to do so by citing the opinions expressed by the Scientific Committee of the World Federation for Mental Health in the monograph, *Mental Health and Value Systems,* edited by Kenneth Soddy.

In the first chapter, the authors candidly acknowledge "that mental health is associated with principles dependent upon the prevailing religion or ideology of the community concerned."[30]

There then follows a review of the various concepts of mental health proposed by different workers. For example, in Soddy's opinion, "A healthy person's response to life is without strain; his ambitions are within the scope of practical realization. . . ."[31] While in the opinion of a colleague whose view he cites, mental health "demands good interpersonal relations with oneself, with others, and with God"[32]—a definition that neatly places all atheists in the class of the mentally sick.

The authors consider the vexing problem of the relation between social adaptation and mental health. They succeed admirably in evading the problem that they claim to be tackling: "[M]ental health and social adaptation are not identical. . . . [This] can be illustrated by the fact that few people would regard a person who had become better adjusted as a result of leaving home and moving into a different society as having thereby become mentally healthy. . . . In the past, and still today in some societies, adaptation to society has tended to be highly valued . . . as a sign of mental health; and failure to adapt has been even more strongly regarded as a sign of mental ill-health. . . . There are occasions and situations in which, from the point of view of mental health, rebellion and non-conformity may be far more important than social adaptation."[33] But no criteria are given for distinguishing, "from the point of view of mental health," the situations to which we ought to conform from those against which we ought to rebel.

There is much more of this kind of sanctimonious foolishness. Thus we are told, "While it is unlikely that agreement could be reached on the proposition that all 'bad' people are mentally unhealthy, it might be possible to agree that no 'bad' person could be said to have the highest possible level of mental health, and that many 'bad' people are mentally unhealthy."[34] The problems of who is to decide who the "bad" people are, and by what criteria they are to decide, are glossed over. This evasion of the reality of conflicting ethics in the world as it exists is the most outstanding feature of this study. Perhaps one of the aims of propounding a fuzzy, yet comprehensive, mental health ethic is to maintain this denial. Indeed, the true goal of the community psychiatrist seems to be to replace a clear political vocabulary with an obscure psychiatric semantic, and a pluralistic system of moral values with a singularistic mental health ethic. Here is an example of the way this is accomplished:

"Our view is that the assumption of an attitude of superiority by one social group towards another is not conducive to the mental health of either group."[35] Some simplistic comments about the Negro problem in America then follow. No doubt, the sentiment here expressed is admirable. But the real problems of psychiatry are bound up not with abstract groups but with concrete individuals. Yet nothing is said about actual relations between people—for example, between adults and children, doctors and patients, experts and clients; and how, in these various situations, the attainment of a relationship that is both egalitarian and functional requires the utmost skill and effort of all concerned (and may, in some cases, be impossible to realize).

Self-revealing as the mental health ethicist is when he discusses mental health and illness, his moral stance is even clearer when he discusses psychiatric treatment. Indeed, the promoter of mental health now emerges as a social engineer on the grand scale: he will be satisfied with nothing less than gaining license to export his own ideology to a world market.

The authors begin their discussion of the promotion of mental health by noting the "resistances" against it: "The principles underlying success in attempts to alter cultural conditions *in the interest of mental health,* and the hazards of such attempts, are very important considerations for practical mental health work. ... The introduction of change in a community may be subject to conditions not unlike those which obtain in the case of *the child ...*" (italics added).[36] We recognize here the familiar medical-psychiatric model of human relations: the client is like the ignorant child who must be "protected," if need be autocratically and without his consent, by the expert, who is like the omnicompetent parent.

The mental health worker who subscribes to this point of view and engages in this kind of work adopts a condescending attitude toward his (unwilling) clients: he regards them, at best, as stupid children in need of education, and, at worst, as evil criminals in need of correction. All too often he seeks to impose value change through fraud and force, rather than through truth and example. In brief, he does not practice what he preaches. The egalitarian-loving attitude toward one's fellow man, which the mental health worker is so eager to export to the "psychiatrically underdeveloped" areas of the world, seems to be in rather short supply everywhere. Or are we to overlook the relations in the United States between white and black, or psychiatrist and involuntary patient?

The authors are not wholly oblivious of these difficulties. But they seem to think it sufficient to acknowledge their awareness of such problems. For example, after commenting on the similarities between Chinese brainwashing and involuntary psychiatric treatment, they write:

"The term brain-washing has ... been applied with unfortunate connotations to psychotherapeutic practice *by those who are hostile to it.* We consider that the lesson of this needs to be taken to heart by all who are responsible for securing psychiatric treatment of non-volitional patients. The use of compulsion or deceit will almost certainly *appear, to those who are unfriendly to or frightened of* the aims of psychotherapy, to be wicked" (italics added).[37]

The "benevolent" despot, whether political or psychiatric, does not like to have his benevolence questioned. If it is, he resorts to the classic tactic of the oppressor: he tries to silence his critic, and, if this fails, he tries to degrade him. The psychiatrist accomplishes this by calling those who disagree with him "hostile" or "mentally ill." Here we are told that if a person admits to the similarities between brain-washing and involuntary psychiatric treatment he is, *ipso facto, hostile* to psychotherapy.

The statement about "the lesson ... to be taken to heart by all who are *responsible* for securing psychiatric treatment of non-volitional patients" [italics added] requires special comment. The language used implies that involuntary mental patients exist in nature—whereas, in fact, they are created, largely by psychiatrists. Thus, after raising the vexing problem of involuntary psychiatric treatment, the authors fail to deal with it in a clear and forthright manner; instead, they impugn the emotional health and moral intentions of those who would dare to look at the problem critically.

This antagonism to a critical examination of his doctrines and methods may be necessary for the mental health worker, just as it is for the missionary or the politician: the aim of each is to conquer souls or minds, not to understand human problems. Let us not forget the dangers of trying to understand another person: the effort invites disproof of one's views and questioning of one's beliefs. The thoughtful person who is content to teach by the example of his own conduct must always be ready to acknowledge error and to change his ways. But this is not what the mental health worker wants: he does not want to change his ways, but those of others.

In an analysis of the mental hygiene movement written nearly thirty years ago, Kingsley Davis has suggested this and more. Commenting on the "family clinic," Davis observed that such agencies offer not medical treatment but moral manipulation: "Before one can cure such patients, one must alter their purpose; in short, one must operate, not on their anatomy, but on their system of values."[38] The trouble is, of course, that people usually do not want to *alter* their goals—they want to *attain* them. As a result, "Only those clients whose ends correspond to socially sanctioned values may be expected to come voluntarily to such a clinic. Other troubled persons, whose wishes are opposed to accepted values, will stay away; they can be brought in only through force or fraud."[39] Nor does Davis shirk from stating what many know but few dare articulate—namely, that ". . . many clients are lured to family clinics by misrepresentation."[40] Similarly, many more are lured to state mental hospitals and community-sponsored clinics. Community psychiatry thus emerges, in my opinion at least, as a fresh attempt to revitalize and expand the old mental hygiene industry.

First, there is a new advertising campaign: mental health education is an effort to lure unsuspecting persons into becoming clients of the community mental health services. Then, having created a demand—or, in this case, perhaps merely the appearance of one—the industry expands: this takes the form of steadily increasing expenditures for existing mental hospitals and clinics and for creating new, more highly automated factories, called "community mental health centers."

Before concluding this review of the ethics of mental health work, I want to comment briefly on the values advocated by the authors of *Mental Health and Value Systems*.

They promote change as such; its direction is often left unspecified. "The success of mental health promotion depends partly upon the creation of a climate favorable to change and a belief that change is desirable and possible."[41] They also emphasize the need to scrutinize certain "unproven assumptions"; none of these, however, pertains to the nature of mental health work. Instead, they list as unproven assumptions such ideas as ". . . the mother is always the best person to have charge of her own child."[42]

I believe that we ought to object to all this on basic logical and moral grounds: if moral values are to be discussed and promoted, they ought to be considered for what they are—moral values, not health values. Why? Because moral values are, and must be, the legitimate concern of everyone and fall under the special competence of no particular group; whereas health values (and especially their technical implementation) are, and must be, the concern mainly of experts on health, especially physicians.

V

Regardless of what we call it, mental health today is a big business. This is true in every modern society, whatever its political structure. It is impossible, therefore, to comprehend the struggle between individualistic and collectivistic values in psychiatry without a clear understanding of the social organization of mental health care.

Surprising as it may seem, in the United States 98 per cent of the care for the hospitalized mentally ill is provided by federal, state, and county governments.[43] The situation in Great Britain is similar. In the Soviet Union the figure is, of course, 100 per cent.

To be sure, this is not the whole picture for the United States or Great Britain. Private practice is still what the term implies: private. Yet this does not mean that psychiatric inpatient care is paid for by public funds, and psychiatric outpatient care by private funds. Outpatient services are financed both privately and publicly. Including all types of care, it has been estimated that "about 65% of all the treatment of mental patients goes on in tax supported services, and 35% in private and voluntary services."[44]

The implications of the vast and expanding involvement of the government in mental health care have, I think, been insufficiently appreciated. Moreover, whatever problems stem from government control of mental hospital care, these difficulties are connected with a logically antecedent problem: What is the aim of the care provided? It does not help to say that it is to transform the mentally sick into the mentally healthy. We have seen that the terms "mental health" and "mental sickness" designate ethical values and social performances. The mental hospital system thus serves, however covertly, to promote certain values and performances, and to suppress others. Which values are promoted and which suppressed depends, of course, on the nature of the society sponsoring the "health" care.

Again, these points are not new. Similar views have been voiced by others. Davis observed that the prospective clients of family clinics "are told in one way or another, through lectures, newspaper publicity, or discreet announcement, that the clinic exists for the purpose of helping individuals out of their troubles; whereas it really exists for the purpose of helping the established social order. Once lured to the clinic, the individual may suffer further deception in the form of propaganda to the effect that his own best interest lies in doing the thing he apparently does not want to do, as if a man's 'best interest' could be judged by anything else than his own desires."[45]

Because of the involuntary character of this kind of clinic or hospital, it follows, according to Davis (and I agree with him), that the service "must find support through subsidy (philanthropic or governmental) rather than through profit from fees. Furthermore, since its purpose is identified with the community at large rather than the person it serves, and since it requires the use of force or misrepresentation to carry out this purpose, it must function as an arm of the law and government. We do not permit the use of force and fraud to individuals in their private capacity. ... In order, therefore, to settle familial conflicts by enforcing social dictates, a family clinic must in the long run be clothed with the power or at least the mantle of some state-authorized institution for the exercise of systematic deception, such as the church."[46]

Could the community support a clinic devoted to promoting the best interests of the client, rather than of the community? Davis considered this possibility, and concluded that it could not. For, if this kind of clinic is to exist, then, "like the other kind, [it] must use force and deception—not on the client, but on the community. It must lobby in legislative halls, employ political weapons, and above all deny publicly its true purpose."[47] (We have seen organized American psychoanalysis do just this.)[48]

Davis is clear about the basic alternatives that psychiatry must face, but that it refuses to face: "The individualistic clinic would accept the standard of its client. The other kind of clinic would accept the standard of society. In practice only the latter is acceptable, because the state is clothed with the power to use force and fraud."[49] Insofar as family clinics or other kinds of mental health facilities try to render services of both kinds, "they are trying to ride two horses headed in opposite directions."[50]

Comparison of the care provided by mental hospitals in Russia and America supports the contention that the values and performances that psychiatry promotes or suppresses are related to the society sponsoring the psychiatric service. The proportion of physicians and hospital beds to population is about the same in both countries. However, this similarity is misleading. In the Soviet Union, there are about 200,000 psychiatric hospital beds; in the United States, about 750,000. Accordingly, "11.2% of all hospital beds in the Soviet Union [are] allocated to psychiatric patients, compared with 46.4% in the USA."[51]

This difference is best accounted for by certain social and psychiatric policies that encourage mental hospitalization in America, but discourage it in Russia. Moreover, the Soviets' main emphasis in psychiatric care is enforced work, whereas ours is enforced idleness; they compel psychiatric patients to produce, whereas we compel them to consume. It seems improbable that these "therapeutic" emphases should be unrelated to the chronic labor shortage in Russia, and the chronic surplus here.

In Russia, "work therapy" differs from plain work in that the former is carried out under the auspices of a psychiatric institution, the latter under the auspices of a factory or farm. Furthermore, as we saw in the case of Iosif Brodsky, the Russian criminal is sentenced to work—not to idleness (or make-work), like his American counterpart. All this stems from two basic sources: first, from the Soviet sociopolitical theory that holds that "productive work" is necessary and good for both society and the individual; second, from the Soviet socioeconomic fact that in a system of mammoth bureaucracies (lacking adequate checks and balances) more and more people are needed to do less and less work. Thus, the Soviets have a chronic labor shortage.

Consistent with these conditions, the Russians try to keep people at their jobs, rather than put them in mental hospitals. If a person is no longer tolerated at his job, he is made to work in "psychiatric outpatient clinics . . . where patients [can] spend the entire day at work. . . ."[52] In the 1930s, during the heyday of Stalinism, there developed an "uncritical infatuation with work therapy," as a result of which "the hospitals came to resemble industrial plants."[53]

It is evident that the distinction, in Russia, between

work therapy and plain work is of the same kind as the distinction, in the United States, between confinement in a hospital for the criminally insane and imprisonment in jail. Many of the Soviet hospital shops, we learn, "settle down to operate like regular factory units, keeping their mildly disabled but productive patients there for interminable periods, paying them regular wages while they travel daily back and forth to their homes as if they had permanent jobs. ... Instances have been reported where the sheltered workshops have been exploited by their managers for private gain...."[54]

In the United States, the government does not usually own or control the means of production. The manufacture of goods and the provision of (most) services is in the hands of private individuals or groups. If the government should have persons under its care produce goods or provide services, it would create a problem of competition with private enterprise. This problem first arose in connection with prisons and now faces us in connection with mental health facilities. The stockholders of General Motors Corporation (or its employees) would be less than happy if the United States Government were to have the inmates of federal prisons manufacture automobiles. Thus, prisoners in America are reduced to making license plates, and mental patients, to mopping floors or working in the kitchen or back ward of the hospital.

The point I wish to make is simple: unlike in Russia, the major socioeconomic problem in the United States is an over-abundance, not a scarcity, of consumer goods; likewise, we have an excess, not a shortage, of productive manpower. The result is our well-known chronic unemployment, which rarely dips below 5 per cent of the labor force (without including many elderly persons capable of working). Accordingly, in American mental hospitals, meaningful and productive work is discouraged and, if need be, prevented by force. Instead of defining forced labor as therapy—as do the Soviets—we define forced idleness as therapy. The only work permitted (or encouraged) is labor necessary to maintain the hospital plant and services, and, even in this category, only such work as is considered non-competitive with private enterprise.

As I suggested some time ago,[55] in the United States mental hospitalization serves a twofold socioeconomic function. First, by defining people in mental hospitals as unfit for work (and often preventing them from working even after their discharge), the mental health care system serves to diminish our national pool of unemployment; large numbers of people are classified as mentally ill rather than as socially incompetent or unemployed. Second, by creating a vast organization of psychiatric hospitals and affiliated institutions, the mental health care system helps to provide employment; indeed, the number of psychiatric and parapsychiatric jobs thus created is staggering. As a result, major cutbacks in the expenditures of the mental health bureaucracy threaten the same kind of economic dislocation as do cutbacks in the expenditures of the defense establishment and are, perhaps, equally "unthinkable."

It seems to me, therefore, that contrary to the oft-repeated propaganda about the high cost of mental illness, we have a subtle economic stake in perpetuating, and even increasing, such "illness." Faced as we are with overproduction and underemployment, we can evidently afford the "cost" of caring for hundreds of thousands of "mental patients" and their dependents. But can we afford the "cost" of not caring for them, and thus adding to the ranks of the unemployed not only the so-called mentally ill, but also the people who now "treat" them and do "research" on them?

Whatever the ostensible aims of community psychiatry may be, its actual operations are likely to be influenced by socioeconomic and political considerations and facts such as I have discussed here.

VI

Psychiatry is a moral and social enterprise. The psychiatrist deals with problems of human conduct. He is, therefore, drawn into situations of conflict—often between the individual and the group. If we wish to understand psychiatry, we cannot avert our eyes from this dilemma: we must know whose side the psychiatrist takes—the individual's or the group's.

Proponents of the mental health ideology describe the problem in different terms. By not emphasizing conflicts between people, they avoid enlisting themselves explicitly as the agents of either the individual or the group. As they prefer to see it, instead of promoting the interests of one or another party or moral value, they promote "mental health."

Considerations such as these have led me to conclude that the concept of mental illness is a betrayal of common sense and of an ethical view of man. To be sure, whenever we speak of a concept of man, our initial problem is one of definition and philosophy: What do we mean by man? Following in the tradition of individualism and rationalism, I hold that a human being is a person to the extent that he makes free, uncoerced choices. Anything that increases his freedom, increases his manhood; anything that decreases his freedom, decreases his manhood.

Progressive freedom, independence, and responsibility lead to being a man; progressive enslavement, dependence, and irresponsibility, to being a thing. Today it is inescapably clear that, regardless of its origins and aims, the concept of mental illness serves to enslave man. It does so by permitting—indeed commanding— one man to impose his will on another.

We have seen that the purveyors of mental health care, especially when such care is provided by the government, are actually the purveyors of the moral and socioeconomic interests of the state. This is hardly surprising. What other interests could they represent? Surely not those of the so-called patient, whose interests are often antagonistic to those of the state. In this way, psychiatry—now proudly called "community psychiatry"—becomes largely a means of controlling the individual. In a mass society, this is best accomplished by recognizing his existence only as a member of a group, never as an individual.

The danger is clear, and has been remarked on by

others. In America, when the ideology of totalitarianism is promoted as fascism or communism, it is coldly rejected. However, when the same ideology is promoted under the guise of mental health care, it is warmly embraced. It thus seems possible that where fascism and communism have failed to collectivize American society, the mental health ethic may yet succeed.

REFERENCES

1. See Szasz, T. S.: *The Myth of Mental Illness: Foundations of a Theory of Personal Conduct* (New York: Hoeber-Harper, 1961).
2. Popper, K. R.: *The Open Society and Its Enemies* (Princeton, N.J.: Princeton University Press, 1950).
3. Fromm, E.: *Escape from Freedom* (New York: Rinehart, 1941).
4. Quoted in *The New York Times,* August 31, 1964, p. 8.
5. "The trial of Iosif Brodsky: A transcript." *The New Leader,* 47: 6-17 (August 31), 1964.
6. Ibid., p. 14.
7. For a comparison of Soviet criminal law and American mental hygiene law, see Szasz, T. S.: *Law, Liberty, and Psychiatry: An Inquiry into the Social Uses of Mental Health Practices* (New York: Macmillan, 1963), pp. 218-21.
8. "The trial of Iosif Brodsky," op. cit., p. 14.
9. See Szasz, *Law, Liberty, and Psychiatry, supra,* Chap. 17.
10. Tarsis, V.: *Ward 7: An Autobiographical Novel,* transl. by Katya Brown (London and Glasgow: Collins and Harvill, 1965).
11. "Roche Report: Community psychiatry and mental hospitals." *Frontiers of Hospital Psychiatry,* I:1-2 & 9 (November 15), 1964.
12. Ibid., p. 2.
13. Ibid.
14. Ibid.
15. Ibid., p. 9.
16. Ibid.
17. For further discussion, see Szasz, T. S.: "Whither psychiatry?" This volume, pp. 218-45.
18. Kennedy, J. F.: *Message from the President of the United States Relative to Mental Illness and Mental Retardation,* February 5, 1963; 88th Cong., First Sess., House of Representatives, Document No. 58; reprinted in *Amer. J. Psychiatry,* 120:729-37 (Feb.), 1964, p. 730.
19. Caplan, G.: *Principles of Preventive Psychiatry* (New York: Basic Books, 1964), p. 3.
20. Ibid.
21. Quoted in Gorman, M.: "Psychiatry and public policy." *Amer. J. Psychiatry,* 122:55-60 (Jan.), 1965, p. 56.
22. Parkinson, C. N.: *Parkinson's Law and Other Studies in Administration* [1957] (Boston: Houghton Mufflin Co., 1962).
23. Caplan, op. cit., p. 56.
24. Ibid., p. 59.
25. Ibid., pp. 62-63.
26. Ibid., p. 65.

27. Ibid.

28. Ibid., p. 79.

29. See Szasz, *The Myth of Mental Illness, supra;* also "The myth of mental illness." This volume, pp. 12-24, and "The rhetoric of rejection." This volume, pp. 49-68.

30. Soddy, K., ed.: *Cross-Cultural Studies in Mental Health: Identity, Mental Health, and Value Systems* (Chicago: Quadrangle, 1962), p. 70.

31. Ibid., p. 72.

32. Ibid., p. 73.

33. Ibid., pp. 75-76.

34. Ibid., p. 82.

35. Ibid., p. 106.

36. Ibid., p. 173.

37. Ibid., p. 186.

38. Davis, K.: "The application of science to personal relations: A critique of the family clinic idea." *Amer. Sociological Rev.,* 1:236-47 (April), 1936, p. 238.

39. Ibid., p. 241.

40. Ibid.

41. Soddy, op. cit., p. 209.

42. Ibid., p. 208.

43. Blain, D.: "Action in mental health: Opportunities and responsibilities of the private sector of society." *Amer. J. Psychiatry,* 121:422-27 (Nov.), 1964, p. 425.

44. Ibid.

45. Davis, op. cit., pp. 241-42.

46. Ibid., pp. 242-43.

47. Ibid., p. 243.

48. See Szasz, T. S.: "Psychoanalysis and taxation: A contribution to the rhetoric of the disease concept in psychiatry." *Amer. J. Psychotherapy,* 18:635-43 (Oct.), 1964; "A note on psychiatric rhetoric." *Amer. J. Psychiatry,* 121:1192-93 (June), 1965.

49. Davis, op. cit., p. 244.

50. Ibid., p. 245.

51. Wortis, J. and Freundlich, D.: "Psychiatric work therapy in the Soviet Union," *Amer. J. Psychiatry,* 121:123-25 (Aug.), 1964, p. 123.

52. Ibid.

53. Ibid., p. 124.

54. Ibid., p. 127.

55. Szasz, T. S.: "Review of *The Economics of Mental Illness,* by Rashi Fein (New York: Basic Books, 1958)." *AMA Archives of General Psychiatry,* 1:116-18 (July), 1959.

Part VI
Role Diffusion

ROLE DIFFUSION

"Role Diffusion" has three aspects. 1) Professionals perform functions in community mental health for which they are not trained, e.g., a psychiatrist does community organization work. 2) Important mental health functions are carried out by people who ordinarily are not thought of as being in the mental health field. For example, mental health functions may involve "gatekeepers" (police, storekeepers, lawyers, general practitioners, etc.), volunteers, patient' families, and patients themselves. 3) The role of "patient" or "person in need of help" is not restricted. "Role Diffusion" is the opposite of the system of highly differentiated tasks for the different mental health disciplines and diagnostic categorization of patients for the selection process. It implies that all mental health professionals can carry out most mental health functions, that people not in the mental health field can be trained to carry out certain functions, and that all people, regardless of age, diagnosis, or severity of emotional problems, can receive help.

Advocates of this point of view see it as being democratic, just, and an answer to the limitations of professional manpower. Some advocates believe that "Role Diffusion" yields certain advantages even when the scarcity of professional manpower is not a problem. A situation in which mental health professionals can fill in for each other offers more flexibility and allows these professionals to achieve a greater understanding of each other's role. Some functions may even be done best by a nonprofessional. For example, a person who has lived in the ghetto may be able to communicate more effectively with other ghetto residents.

Opponents of this point of view believe that acquiring mental health expertise is a long, arduous road that requires long training and cannot be shared indiscriminately. There are great risks in assigning nonprofessionals to do psychotherapy, community organization, etc. Even seemingly simpler tasks such as home visits may take more skill than a well-meaning but untrained volunteer may have. Furthermore, the different mental health disciplines have each developed their own expertise and the best use of their time is achieved by involving them in tasks for which they have been specially trained. While a psychiatrist may be assigned to do community organization in a community mental health center, he will probably not do as well at this as a trained social worker, and the time he spends in community organization might be better spent in tasks in which he is skilled and for which there is great demand.

Dr. George W. Albee argues that scarcity and constraints of mental health manpower require role diffusion. Dr. Albee is Professor of Psychology at the University of Vermont. Formerly he was president of the American Psychological Association and Chairman, Department of Psychology, Case Western Reserve University. Dr. Albee has written extensively on mental health manpower problems and was director of the Task Force on Manpower for the Joint Commission on Mental Illness and Health during 1957-1959.

Mrs. Shirley Cooper is Chief Psychiatric Social Worker, Department of Psychiatry, Mount Zion Hospital in San Francisco, and Associate Professor, San Francisco State College. She has published extensively on trends in social work, supervision and training, and community mental health. She serves as a consultant to a number of social agencies and is on the board of directors of the American Orthopsychiatric Association. In her article on "Role Diffusion" she questions many of the assumptions of this concept and thoughtfully considers its many ramifications and the problems it entails.

THE SICKNESS MODEL OF MENTAL DISORDER MEANS A DOUBLE STANDARD OF CARE*

George W. Albee

Let me begin by arguing that the explanatory *model* used to account for disturbed and deviant human behavior determines the kind of *institutions* which society supports to provide intervention, and the nature of these institutions in turn determines the *kind of manpower* required for their staffing.

The explanatory model occupying the center of the stage today insists on the fiction that "mental illness is an illness like any other." It trims the stage with institutional trappings of sickness, beds, hospitals, and clinics. As a consequence, our manpower problems are defined as shortages of medical and paramedical professionals, which include the four major actors in the drama—the psychiatrist, clinical psychologist, psychiatric social worker, and psychiatric nurse. The bit players, or extras, we are seeking in large numbers include all the ancillary paramedical professionals needed to fill the depleted ranks in our "treatment institutions."

There is an everwidening gap between the growing manpower needs of our tax-supported treatment institutions and the shrinking supply of high-level professional workers. Partly this is due to an unwillingness to forego the benefits of status agency or private practice to take

* Reprinted from *Michigan Mental Health Research Bulletin,* Winter 1979, Vol. IV, No. 1., pp. 5-17, with permission of author and editor.

underpaid jobs in public agencies serving those most in need of help. As a result there is a great deal of talk today about training a new group of nonprofessionals, or semi-professional people, to staff the places serving primarily the numerous emotionally-distressed poor. This third-rate idea, combined with a large dose of expert public relations, has almost convinced the public that there will soon be enough intervention to go around. Many people actually believe that a large number of housewives actually are being trained to be counselors, that hundreds of storefront intervention centers already exist, and that highly successful intervention is being accomplished in the new comprehensive mental health centers. Actually, this whole show is going to fold in Boston, long before it reaches the Big Time!

What is required in this field is a whole reconceptualization of causation. Once the *sickness model* is replaced with a more valid *social-learning* explanation (which attributes most emotional disturbance to the dehumanized environment rather than to biological defect) there will follow a redefinition of intervention institutions as re-educational or rehabilitative centers which will call for a very different sort of manpower.

I want to develop the argument that this reconceptualization will lead to the establishment of centers staffed primarily by people educated at the bachelors level or less, with nursing, education, and social work as strong contenders for responsibility and leadership.

A GLOOMY FORECAST

One of the several major myths which we must abandon before we can make any progress in closing the manpower gap suggests that somehow, someday, we will have enough traditional mental health professionals, and therefore, the need for nonprofessional, or middle-level, mental health workers is a temporary situation. This myth leads to all sorts of inconsistent behavior in approaching the training of these people. We hesitate to change our civil service requirements. We even fear that if we train *too* many they may organize, take over, and shut us out. The latter situation may come to pass, but we should welcome it.

Actually, there is *no* chance that psychiatry and psychology, as these disciplines are now defined, will ever provide the necessary amount of manpower for effective intervention.[1] Indeed, the number of people in these precious, highly-specialized disciplines will decrease rather than increase over the next couple of decades in proportion to population.

Let us take the field of psychiatry as an example. During the past two decades, as a result of an enormous financial investment in psychiatric training by the National Institute of Mental Health, together with the massive importation of foreign physicians, the membership of the American Psychiatric Association has quadrupled. But during this same period, *the number of psychiatrists employed in tax-supported mental institutions has declined in absolute numbers!*

Today we have some 2,000 psychiatric clinics scattered throughout our land. However, more than two-thirds of these clinics do not have a single full-time psychiatrist on their staff! Obviously something at least equal to the miracle of the loaves and fishes will be required to staff the 2,000 comprehensive community mental health centers that are to be built by NIMH in the next decade.

Nor would a crash program to increase the number of psychiatrists trained have much effect. In the first place, the long-time policy of the American Medical Association to hold down medical school enrollments has resulted in a shortage of physicians which grows steadily greater. Each year we are at least 3,000 new M.D.'s behind the number that would be required simply to hold our own in ratio of physicians to population. And psychiatry must draw most of it recruits from the same limited pool where all the other medical specialties, equally hungry for residents, are seeking their neophytes.[2]

But suppose by some magic we could double the output of our medical schools and thereby double the number of young M.D.'s going into psychiatric residencies. It would still be a hopeless situation. When we look at the *distribu-*

tion of psychiatrists we find that more than 50 percent of our nation's total are to be found in the five favored (is that the right word?) states of Massachusetts, Pennsylvania, New York, Illinois, and California. Within these states, of course, the psychiatrists are concentrated in suburbia, where 80 per cent of psychiatry is practiced in private offices (with a white, middle-class, largely female, non-Catholic clientele.)[2]

I will not take time to recite comparable statistics for other mental health professions except to make it quite clear that I have no hidden agenda which intends somehow to advance *psychology* in the care-delivery field. Let me tell you quite bluntly that clinical psychology is going to disappear from the marketplace for the next 10-20 years, as the relative handful of people we are able to produce is recruited into academic teaching where serious shortages are developing, and where the psychologist is not a second-class citizen but breathes the air of academic freedom. It is also worth noting that there are 20 vacant positions for every graduate of social work, and that qualified psychiatric nurses are as close to extinction as the blue whale.

TRAINING FOR NEW OR OLD?

Psychiatrist Moody Bettis[3] recently raised the crucial question when he asked whether solutions to "the manpower problem" involve training people for where we are trying to go, or for where we have been! Do we want to train people for new community programs or old institutional programs? Do we want to reconsider the adequacy of many of the institutions of the past or continue to regard them as somehow sacred and above change?

Generally we think of action programs aimed at reducing emotional disturbance in our society in terms that have traditionally been associated with institutional programs. We think of highly trained mental health professionals—medical and paramedical—intervening on a one-to-one basis in some specific physical place (clinic or hospital) in the community. It is very difficult for us to get over our belief that the things we have been doing for so long (and so ineffectively) in our clinics and public hospitals are wrong or worthless. Many programs achieve sanctification through use, a sacred cow status which requires that they continue to be used in the community.

Perhaps the most entrenched and pervasive attitude that influences our thinking about approaches to the preparation of new mental health workers has it that they are to be employed in existing agencies and institutions. Most of the accounts I have read of new training programs for various new kinds of workers imply that they will be used to help relieve senior people—"under careful supervision." The implication is quite clear that many of these workers are to fit into the conventional care-delivery structures as "assistants."

Behind this assumption, of course, lurks that old devil, the *sickness model*. Without beating further what is at least a sickening horse, if not a dead one, I think it is still important to point out that our professions' adherence to the sickness explanation of disturbed behavior ("mental illness is an illness like any other") puts us into a Procrustean model which binds us to hospitals (Procrustean beds?) and clinics as our primary intervention centers.

I would emphasize that a significant component of the enthusiasm for training middle-level-workers originates among those seeking a solution for the glaringly inadequate staffing of our tax-supported public facilities. These new people are sought to staff, primarily, state hospitals, county-run child centers, retardation centers, etc. A cynical way of viewing this situation would be to suggest that there will always be just enough high-class, highly-trained mental health professionals to work in psychiatric wards in general hospitals, university hospitals and clinics, and in high prestige agencies, as well as private practice. We have known for years that the shortages become more and more acute in the facilities that serve the poor—the public agencies, public clinics and public hospitals. Recently Mike Gorman[8] pointed out that in well over a third of the state hospitals in this country, little or no psychiatric time is available. My guess is that even this is a minimum estimate.

THE ROLE OF THE CCMHC

The Comprehensive Community Mental Health Centers (CCMHC) movement, originally conceived as a shining hope for the poor, and described as small intensive community-based centers in the heart of our cities, where the largest number of disturbed people is to be found, has now been captured and used to increase the resources of middle-class serving general hospitals. The regulations for CCMHC's were written in such a way that a general hospital with a psychiatric unit could qualify for construction funds if it agreed to use even 10% of the beds for the indigent, beds newly built with tax dollars. This means that in a majority of the CCMHC's now being built in general hospitals, the poor will be largely excluded.

As a matter of fact this probably also means that middle level mental health workers will be excluded too. General hospitals are not known for their eagerness to hire salaried people whose services are not billable. Indeed, most CCMHC's get by with a very minimum of psychological and social work help.[7] The whole emphasis in the funding of the CCMHC program has been on the granting of construction funds to add beds. General hospitals make their income from the use of beds, and the fortunate few psychiatrists who control bed privileges have a good thing. Does this sound cynical? Listen to the psychiatrist-director of the Los Angeles County Department of Mental Health (Harry R. Brickman, M.D.):

> Those responsible for mental health programs must soon decide whether they wish to build a vast new social machinery which will paradoxically "create" illness under the banner of health or whether they wish to grasp a real opportunity to help build a more humanistic community which is emotionally nutritive and which is increasingly tolerant and constructively helpful to social deviation in all forms.[6]

Dr. Brickman goes on to argue that the CCMHC's must not be considered an end in themselves. Rather they should be a means toward achieving a better and more humanistic society with intervention primarily carried out "by non-psychiatric agents." There is little evidence that this will happen.

Somehow as our society becomes more dehumanized, more consumption-oriented and more and more inbred with the philosophy: "I'll get mine, Jack," the more we seem to need "helping" professionals. For most of the world the mental health professions are unknown or unwanted. The Peace Corps does not receive requests for psychiatrists or clinical psychologists. In societies where families, neighborhood, religious institutions, and tradition provide comfort and support, relationship therapy is unneeded or unknown. It is only as we move toward a society of strangers, highly mobile, without roots, with little tradition, and few stable relationships that we develop a market for "the purchase of friendship" (William Schofield's apt name for psychotherapy). I would not argue against the fact that there are large numbers of lonely and lost people in our society who need help. It is simply that we can never solve our human problems by trying to put these people into hospitals or clinics, by calling them patients, and by giving them individual treatment by our traditional methods.

EFFECTIVE INTERVENTION

From one perspective the most effective interventionists responsible for increasing and improving the mental health of millions of citizens need not be conventionally trained mental health workers at all. If we could reach newspaper publishers, TV advertisers, and disc jockeys—who have more input than most professional organizations—we might cause really effective intervention.

Let me suggest an example of what I have in mind.

Recently two Black psychiatrists, Grier and Cobbs,[9] spelled out in searing and stark detail the tragic consequences of our racist white society's behavior for the mental health of Black citizens.

Millions of Black children grow up in a racist white society which thoughtlessly and chauvinistically equates attractiveness in children and adults with fair, straight hair and regular features. The damaged self-concepts and damaged interpersonal relationships which result for Black children might be eliminated very quickly if, for example, the federal government (Federal Communications Commission) were to order that at least 20% of all commercial advertisements use Black models; that all actors in television dramas be employed without regard to skin color, and that our vast communication industry be rewarded with tax credits for effective techniques it develops to transmit the message that beauty and attractiveness can take many colors and forms.

As a matter of fact I find myself continually falling into the bad habit of thinking our mental health problems involve primarily schizophrenic and other serious conventional disorders. When I stop to consider, I do *not* believe that the most significant mental health problems of our society today are to be found in the population of our state hospitals, *nor* in the clientele of our outpatient psychiatric clinics, *nor* do I believe that our most serious mental health problems are to be found in the psychiatric wards of our general hospitals.

Our most significant mental health problems exist in middle-class people who rarely end up in a clinic or mental institution. I speak of the white racists identified in the Kerner Report, and their dehumanized fellows—perhaps most of us—who accept institutions that do not strengthen people but dehumanize them. It follows that a significant number of the mental health workers that I believe must be recruited and educated will hardly be identified as such, but rather as a cadre who may provide future leadership in combatting and reducing the amount of dehumanized aggression in our society and in our world, and increasing the amount of responsible human interaction of which humans are capable. These recruits are available in significant numbers in our undergraduate colleges. I believe the Kerner Report is right in reporting white racism to be the major cause of the social unrest in our society. I believe also that we are moving (often with maddening delays and detours), toward an integrated society in which all human beings will be able to live and love more freely. The consequences of achieving such a society, in mental health terms, will far exceed any new treatment techniques, or new psychotropic drug discoveries, or any number of new mental health workers trained as interventionists.

The morally destructive forces in our society—forces that have polluted our environment, destroyed our lakes and streams, deforested our national parks, strip-mined our hills and fields, and turned our cities into a hideous blight—the same forces that have supported meaningless wars and have poured billions down the rat hole of accelerating militarism—they are also responsible for the dehumanization of our social environment. Our society is proselytized and propagandized into thinking that wasteful, meaningless consumption is the highest end of living. We are told that human sexuality is obscene but murder, violence and aggression are entertaining. This obscene philosophy, which negates the importance of social relationships, produces dehumanized and irrational consumers unresponsive or refractory to violence and suffering whose fragmented emotional lives lead increasing numbers to go out of control.

Then the Establishment (the military-industrial complex that President Eisenhower warned us against) proceeds to explain away the increasing social pathology as being a result of individual defect (mental illness is an illness like any other) and escapes responsibility by well-publicized support of biochemical research aimed at discovering "causes and cures."

MOST NEEDED MENTAL HEALTH WORKERS

While a major contribution to the problems in our society originates in white racism, a significant amount of the actual resulting damage is done to the poor and the Black. While we are trying to change the pattern of racist behavior our society must also develop interventionists to ameliorate the damage already done. These interventionists should be drawn largely from the disadvantaged groups themselves. I think they should be essentially BA-level people, and we should make urgent efforts to recruit and train special interventionists from Black and from other disadvantaged groups. It is more and more difficult to separate mental health problems from welfare problems and from educational problems. The most needed middle-level mental health workers may turn out to be specially-selected teachers.

We also need bachelors-level social welfare workers in our public agencies serving the inner-city to do something about such problems as the high rate of "mental deficiency" revealed there by epidemiological studies. Most of these cases of retardation are not due to organic factors but are due to impoverished and demoralized conditions of life. Olshansky[10] studied 1,000 children in Boston whose families were receiving Aid for Dependent Children and discovered that nearly seven per cent were functionally retarded. I believe that social welfare workers and pre-school teachers and visiting nurses (all primarily Black) must be the interventionists until we can reform our cities and eliminate slums and ghettoes.

I am not convinced that we need a new generic, all-purpose, middle-level mental health worker to work in institutions. We need a number of different kinds of mental health workers, trained primarily at the bachelors level, but many of them could develop out of existing professions.

A profession is distinguished from other occupations primarily by the fact that it has *theory* which the aspiring young professional must learn before he begins practice. There is also a sense of lifetime *career choice,* together with the learning of a special language, and ultimate responsibility for the indoctrination of the neophyte. With 40-50 per cent of our college age youngsters enrolled in some kind of higher education, the new mental health workers are going to have to be professionals, or we are not going to recruit them.

One problem arises immediately. Bachelors level professionals have high status when they run their own show. They have low status when they work as assistants to other higher status professionals. Look for example, at the profession of school teaching. It is a nice respectable BA profession because teachers control the schools and have clear cut upwardly mobile paths available. On the other hand, bachelors level people in hospitals are far down the pecking order and are recruited only with difficulty.

I would propose that some of our existing service professions should move quickly to take over or develop their own *care delivery institutions* which they would own and operate. The profession of nursing for example, lacks just one thing to become a major force. It does not have a *care delivery setting* which it owns and controls. Many of the individuals in institutions for the insane and many of those in institutions for the mentally deficient, could be cared for much better in institutions owned and operated by the nursing profession. (So could persons with any of the other chronic organic diseases.) As soon as nursing learns that it must have a setting of its own in which to train its own neophytes, and in which upward bound career patterns are available, I anticipate that nursing will take over and do a much more effective job for the people now cared for in our antiquated state hospital program.

Psychiatric social work is another field that is on the verge of developing an effective independent service delivery system. Social group work is already intervening more frequently and more effectively with the emotionally disturbed poor than any other profession. As soon as psychiatric social workers free themselves from the psychiatric setting and establish their own crisis intervention centers that blend mental health and welfare programs, and that recruit staff from the inner-city people served—or better still as soon as they go to work with group workers in settlement houses located close to where the people are who need help—the sooner good care will be available. In truth, social work is doing most of the psychiatric care in the so-called mental hygiene clinics today. How long will it sit still and see the clinics directed by persons who give a few hours a week and take home high salaries for this limited service to the wrong target groups?

CLERGY, POLICE, AND STUDENTS

In ranging over some of the current literature on mental health training for new groups of professional workers we frequently encounter mental health training for the clergy. Certainly it is true, as we discovered in William Ryan's survey of Boston's mental health services, that the clergy actually provide more counseling and psychotherapy within the American city than do the more traditional mental health professions. (Ryan[11] found that in Boston clergymen were doing more counseling than psychiatrists despite the fact that greater Boston is practically overrun with psychiatrists.) Mental health training for clergymen has usually come to mean training in psycho-dynamics and individual one-to-one intervention. But because most of the important, well-funded and heavily-supported churches and synagogues have moved to suburbia with the rest of the middle-class population, the one-to-one counseling of clergymen tends to be largely limited to middle-class parishioners. In talking with clergymen in my own neighborhood I discover that their counseling is most frequently with people with "drinking problems" and with families trying to cope with pregnant unmarried teenagers.

These clergymen could provide far more significant mental health intervention by leading their congregations toward a firm stand on fair housing and neighborhood integration, perhaps with an emphasis that prejudice and discrimination are grounds for excommunication from the church. This sort of "intervention" will require some significant break-throughs in religious dogma!

Let me cite another existing profession that, with a little change, might become more relevant.

This potential source of new and effective mental health professional workers is the police. I would suggest that we find ways to recruit to the urban police forces some of the same brave and socially motivated young people now attracted to the Peace Corps or the VISTA program. Most police forces are having trouble finding qualified recruits. Instead of such non-constructive activities as many of our young people have engaged in viz-a-viz the police, why not find ways to help them volunteer to spend a few years on the police force trying to help teach the principles of democracy and respect for individual human dignity in this setting.

While on the subject of the police why not use what we know about operants, and reinforcement theory, to single out those policemen who exhibit human relations skills? Policemen who complete training in human relations courses could be given a salary increment, and a further increment or bonus each time they demonstrate that they practice behaviorally what they have learned.

Still another innovative source of people for intervention is the pool of high school students who could be spending time in the elementary school or even in kindergarten classes. In a few pilot projects around the country high school students are spending as much as one day a week working with one, two, or three children in a kindergarten or elementary school in their own district. High school boys, particularly, may be led to discover and experience the universal satisfaction to be derived from a consistent helping relationship with a young child. High school girls, too, may find new skills and satisfactions not available in conventional courses.

Under appropriate reinforcement conditions high school boys and girls can help younger children to learn, but can also serve (self-consciously) as role models. I find no convincing reason why a country that is able to spend $80 million a day in Southeast Asia cannot find a way to pay high school students to work with younger students.

CLOSE STATE MENTAL HOSPITALS

We cannot limit our attention, either, to the pathology of our society and to preventive efforts without paying *some* attention to the unfortunate who have been damaged or destroyed by our system and who now sit out their empty lives in our "state institutions." What is to be done, and who is to do it? Obviously not the present Big Four mental health professions.

Two years ago[1] I suggested that our state hospitals and mental hygiene clinics should be closed and torn down—taken apart piece by piece and stone by stone and then, like the city of Carthage, plowed three feet under and sowed with salt. This proposal was widely reported by the press, and as a consequence I received many letters, some highly supportive and some highly critical. A number of the writers were psychiatrists. Some of them were angry because my suggestion would eliminate their jobs in state hospitals, while others were angry (although they themselves were in private practice and knew relatively little about the state hospitals system) because it was inappropriate for a psychologist to butt into what was essentially a medical problem.

I continue to think the state hospitals should be abandoned, and I cite as supporting participants in this movement two recent presidents of the American Psychiatric Association, Harry C. Solomon[12] and Daniel Blain[5] both of whom suggested in their presidential addresses to their Association that the state hospitals are obsolete and should be eliminated.

The important point is that the state hospitals have come to be a dumping ground for the emotionally disturbed poor, for those who don't have Blue Cross Insurance or some kind of labor union coverage to pay for occupancy of a bed in a general hospital psychiatric ward.

Why bring up this whole matter of state hospitals and the double standard of care? Because much of the demand for the new mental health workers results from the need for such people to work in the state hospitals where medical and paramedical professionals refuse to work. State hospitals and clinics are tax-supported and that makes them socialized medicine and we all know how bad that is! So let's train a host of nonprofessionals to work in these places where we will dump the uninsured poor. Thus we neatly separate our free-enterprise medical intervention with the affluent from our salaried sub-professional services for the poor. Training a corps of sub-professionals to staff the state hospitals would serve to prolong the existence of these antiquated institutions, and perpetuate the double standard of care. One way of blocking this neat but chauvinistic solution would be to close the state hospitals, thereby forcing the community, with good planning, into more effective non-medical programs which might indeed be under the control of BA level professional workers.

If the state hospitals are eliminated, what would happen to all of the present unfortunate inmates, and to those first admission cases who now wind up in the state hospital? It is instructive to look carefully at the poor people in these places now, and those entering them for the first time.

First of all, there is evidence that the unfortunate state hospital inmates are afflicted more by the desocialization that comes from the training these places give them in the role of inmate, than from any real disease process. What has happened for years to people in state hospitals is an almost perfect example of *the self-fulfilling prophecy*. When we admit them we predict that their condition is hopeless, and then we proceed to take away every vestige of humanity, self-respect, and pride, thus creating cases without hope. Then we congratulate ourselves that our original predictions were right.

We know now that at least half the first admissions really do not belong in a "mental hospital." Let me just cite the results of a recent study done by Moody C. Bettis and Robert E. Roberts of the Texas Research Institute of Mental Sciences.[4] Drs. Bettis and Roberts did a systematic study of more than 500 "proposed mentally ill patients" referred to an evaluation center for possible commitment. These people were studied for as much as a week at the center after which they were sent to a local state hospital or discharged back to the community. These scientists found that considerably more than half did *not* need mental hospital commitment, or *would not have* if community services had been available. It turns out that only about one-third of the pre-commitment group should have been put in a mental hospital if *their* need had been the major consideration. As it turns out three-quarters of the group studied were actually committed to the state hospital, because no other solution was available. In a related study the same group of investigators found a significantly large number of persons trapped in the state hospital system who clearly did not belong there but for whom no appropriate intervention was available in the community.

If we were to close the state hospitals, what would happen to the people who presently are entering through their front door?

It is instructive to look at the nature of our first admission group in the state hospitals across the country. As indicated above, the majority of them should not be admitted ever to a state hospital. Half the first admissions are nonpsychotic but represent a mixed group of alcoholics, character disorders, neurotics and lonely people who might be better dealt with in the community.

Of the remaining 50 per cent who are admitted for the first time to state hospitals with the diagnosis of psychosis, half of them are diagnosed "chronic brain syndrome" which means that they are primarily elderly senile individuals who certainly do not deserve the horrible fate of being locked up in a state hospital. Again, better ways of dealing with elderly senile cases can be developed in the community, and in the case of those who require intensive care, general hospitals or nursing homes offer better solutions.

The remaining 25 per cent of first admissions are functionally psychotic. But clearly a significant number of these could be dealt with in foster homes, half-way houses, day or night facilities, and with effective means of community support.

Ordinarily we tell legislators that we need our state hospitals for persons who are "dangerous to themselves or others." But when we look at our first admissions we find that the proportion that is dangerous is a very small number indeed.

We should develop small, tax-supported, comprehensive community mental health centers in the heart of the urban blight. But these centers cannot be medical or paramedical. They may take several forms—some owned and operated by nursing, some by social work, some by special education, and some by new child care professions. Most of the staff should be drawn from the same disadvantaged groups served. The rest of us should be working to bring about the social revolution we need to arrest our nations pell-mell rush toward disaster.

REFERENCES

1. Albee, G. W. 1968. Myths, models, and manpower. Mental Hygiene, 52, 2, April.

2. Albee, G. W. 1967. The relation of conceptual models to manpower needs. In: Cowen, E. L., Gardner, E. A., and Zax, M. (eds.): Emergent Approaches to Mental Health Problems. New York, Appleton-Century-Crofts, 63-73.

3. Bettis, Moody 1969. Personal communication.

4. Bettis, Moody C. and Roberts, Robert E. 1969. Mental health manpower—the dilemma. Mental Hygiene. In Press.

5. Blain, Daniel 1965. Presidential Address. American Journal of Psychiatry.

6. Brickman, Harry R. 1967. Community mental health—means or end? Psychiatric Digest, 28, 43-50.

7. Glasscote, R., et al.: 1964. The Community Mental Health Center. An Analysis of Existing Models. Washington, D.C., The Joint Information Service of the American Psychiatric Association and the National Association for Mental Health.

8. Gorman, Mike 1966. What are the facts about mental illness in the United States. National Committee Against Mental Illness. 66 pp. Pamphlet.

9. Grier, William H. and Cobbs, Price M. 1968. Black Rage. New York: Basic Books.

10. Olshansky, S. and Sternfield, L.A. 1963. A study of suspected cases of mental retardation in families receiving aid to dependent children. American Journal of Public Health, 53, 793.

11. Ryan, W.: 1969. Distress in the City: A Summary Report of the Boston Mental Health Survey. Cleveland: Case Western Reserve University Press.

12. Solomon, Harry 1958. Presidential Address to American Psychiatric Association. American Journal of Psychiatry.

ROLE DIFFUSION—
DILEMMAS AND PROBLEMS*

Shirley Cooper

INTRODUCTION

We live in unsettling times, ambiguous and confusing. Social and ethical certainties vanish into doubt and confusion while revolutionary views are offered with conviction. Change, sometimes propelled by confrontation, creates tensions for professionals, since it demands a review of accepted assumptions and professional definition. Unfortunately, we seem more inclined to advocacy and polemic—the free exchange of ideas and the coexistence of complementary approaches to human problems are hard to retain under the imperative of change. Pressure is couched in such phrases as "innovation," "meaningful response to the community," "relevance," and "serving the unserved." On the one hand, experts are dethroned by the new egalitarianism, while on the other they seek to expand their influence to fields bordering mental health. Mental health perspectives are also influenced by competition for funds and status.

Sharp questions confront the field of mental health: Is mental health a definable field at all, or so intertwined with other aspects of human experience that no boundaries can be set? Are mental health professionals of value or have they impeded progress and service to those in need? Have they outweighed their usefulness by obstinate clinging to tradition and elitist privilege,

* I am indebted to my friends and colleagues Dr. Owen Renik and Dr. Herbert Lau for both contributing and clarifying ideas.

blocking entry of others into their ranks? Is preoccupation with individualism and individual freedom a luxury which obstructs justice for the disadvantaged who must first win their freedom in groups? Has concern for intrapsychic processes retarded the development of important social action? Do those who practice in slow and often tedious ways make service to the many impossible? Are such ways defensible? Since so little is known about effectiveness, are extended training programs for mental health professionals justifiable?

We may not have complete or precise answers to these real and plaguing questions. Yet, if we opt for facile responses because we are overwhelmed by the enormity of the problems, we may hold out false hope and promise.

ROLE DIFFUSION: UNDERLYING PREMISES

Role diffusion describes the result of the "changing functions of the various professional mental health disciplines and . . . the rapidly expanding but uncertain goals of the mental health field in general"[1]. It is occasioned by the increasing variety of contributors to mental health service, most particularly by the use of untrained personnel. Role diffusion is accepted, even welcomed by many mental health professionals whose thinking rests on several premises:

1. We cannot wait many years to train few workers to provide service to a limited handful.

2. Conversely, we must quickly train large numbers of people in extensive methods for reaching the multitude of the formerly unreached.

3. We must yield our maniacal preoccupation with credentials and entry requirements, offering instead learning-by-doing.

4. Ongoing supervision and/or consultation by more expertly trained mental health personnel to new workers will extend the manpower pool.

5. Use of indigenous personnel will bring clients into helpful contact with people closer to their own experience, with the added benefit of reducing communication problems.

6. Consultations will nullify the hazards of brief training.

7. Nonprofessionals can provide effective direct service to those in need, freeing more trained personnel for other tasks.

8. Since their investment in existing social institutions is considerably less intense than arduously trained middle-class experts, nonprofessionals can serve also as vigorous change-agents to alter institutions which adversely affect human beings.

9. New but still uncertain roles properly belong within the domain of mental health.

I will attempt to discuss some of these premises as they relate to issues of professionalism, the boundaries of mental health, clinical practice, and training for professional and nonprofessional mental health workers. First, let me set forth my own views:

1. Although there have been inequities in past practice, new ideas and practices are often instituted for their novelty as much as for their effectiveness.

2. There is a tendency to confuse systems of delivery of care with care itself.

3. There is a growing and hazardous conception that mental health problems and poverty are synonymous. Wealth does not invariably immunize against pathology. nor does poverty inevitably breed it. The middle class is as entitled to service as the formerly unserved poor.

4. We may be developing a newer form of a two-track system in mental health—one for the poor, another for the middle class and the more affluent.

5. Untrained personnel bring special "input" to mental health service, but they may also bring special difficulties which cannot be romanticized away.

6. Social values and professional values are neither synonymous nor completely harmonious. There is value in retaining and recognizing these differences.

7. Consultation and social action cannot replace expert direct mental health services and particularly its psychotherapeutic component.

8. Psychological reality, the domain of mental health, is only one of many different ways of perceiving and explaining the world. While the blurring of different per-

spectives reduces restricting specialization, it carries the danger of destroying clarity of mental health objectives, methods, and review—the very essence of diffusion.

9. Social action to improve the quality of life is essential, but it is not the exclusive province of mental health; to fuse mental health with social action entirely unwittingly undermines democratic processes.

PROFESSIONALISM

"A man's values are like his kidney's; he rarely knows he has any until they are upset. Values become significant when they are challenged. . ."[2].

The issue of role diffusion touches the question of mental health professionalism at its root. If professionalism is a relatively unimportant quality in providing mental health services, then it follows that nonprofessionals can do the job as well, with greater economy and benefit to the community at large and to the consumer in particular. Are we simply in a struggle for position and control in which the "have-nots" challenge the "haves"? Indeed the word "professional" has almost become pejorative, connoting insularity and unconcern with social problems which confront the nation and particularly the disadvantaged. Professionals are indicted for inflating their knowledge and their claim to a special role in dealing with human concerns. Accused of being servants of the establishment, professionals have joined in this questioning, asking themselves whether they have anything valuable to contribute to the central problems of our time. Clearly, professionals themselves are on the defensive.

Questioning about merit did not arise predominantly from the ranks of professionals themselves. It came largely from the outside: from unserved groups who demanded attention; from people clamoring for meaningful work who had heretofore been denied entry into many fields; from the unity and resistance of minority workers who emphasized ethnic concerns and pride, insisting on the superior value of using people of their own group. There is no doubt that professionals have operated in self-serving ways, at times protecting their guild status. To be sure, professionals have clung to a privileged position, irrationally resisting the entry of nonprofessionals. They are threatened in various ways: worried about being supplanted, fearful that the work they do is less skillful than they assumed if others less well trained can do it, uncomfortable about working with people unfamiliar to them. But there is another side. Though forced to reconsider functions, styles of work, and assumptions long taken for granted, professionals are fearful today of being caught with last year's intellectual hemline. They want to be relevant. While they hold ethics which make them responsive to just criticism, they are also concerned for their survival and prone to pressure. These conflicts generate uncertainty and a search for closure. Given these pressures, professionals accept nonprofessional participation in mental health service without sufficient attention to the risks and hazards. Whitehead warns, "to know the truth partially is to distort the universe—an unflinching determination to take the whole evidence into account is the only method of preservation against the fluctuating extremes of fashionable opinion"[3].

Some would argue that since professional performance has not been well documented it is impossible to judge the efficacy of either the professional or the nonprofessional. Granted, the testimony is still not in—nor is it likely to be available soon. Experience with introducing new workers into mental health professions should offer some guides. However, since we cannot rely on hard data, perhaps philosophical concepts can be illuminating. Frankel may here offer some light. He suggests that professionalism, like democracy, cannot be evaluated on performance alone. To indict an idea by its abuse can lead to dangerous distortion. Recognizing that professionals carry out their functions with the sanction of the status quo he disputes that this reveals their true or whole nature as agents of the establishment: "A profession is a meeting place—if you will—a battle ground—between reigning conventions and prejudices, between existing ideologies on the one side, and certain antiseptic concepts on the other. Of these, three are fundamental; they are, indeed, constitutive of the very concept of professionalism. They are 1) The concept of individual merit determined in a neutral fashion; 2) The concept of self-criticism; and 3) The concept of moral impartiality"[4]. Frankel is not naive. He is thoroughly aware of professional limitations. He adds, however, ". . . the cure for intellectual teetotalism is not intellectual alcoholism. I am glad the professions are asking questions about themselves—but I do not welcome the new tide of opinion that calls the very existence of professional values into question; it is fraught with extraordinary dangers—the conflict between the conception of merit that prevails in a given profession and social values emergent in the outside community cannot be resolved by relinquishing the idea of merit or professional competence."[5]

This is the center of a question basic to mental health. The larger community may call us to account for unmet needs and delivery systems of care; though their reactions to the care they receive must be considered, they are far less competent to judge the merit of professional methods. The latter must be fought out within the mental health profession itself. To illustrate: Individuals or groups may, through fear or prejudice, resist hospitalization or surgery, insisting on other methods of treatment for physical disorders. Physicians cannot yield to such pressure. Since mental health methods, often feared, are viewed by the lay population as less specialized and scientific than medical practice, questioning takes on a measure of credability. There is much to debate within the professions; our knowledge about technique is neither complete nor satisfactory. But it will not be augmented or improved by abrogating to the general population the right of disciplined study and criticism.

BOUNDARIES OF MENTAL HEALTH

Role diffusion relates centrally to the issue of defining the boundaries of mental health. A failure to do so can lead to overpromise, inviting disillusion and the creation of more problems than we can solve. These are, of course, of vital consequence. The central issue here is that if we fail to define a legitimate sphere of mental health operations, we can neither describe our tasks nor attempt to train for these in reasonably focal ways.

But is the field definable at all? How can one argue for clarity of role if the tasks to be performed are themselves unclear? Can roles then be assigned to nonprofessionals while others are clearly reserved for professionals?

Recent interest in ecological models has led to the attempt to break down formerly compartmentalized systems of knowledge. Mental health delivery systems reflect this in the development of comprehensive, coordinated, and continuous services. Current recognition that social conditions influence mental health significantly impels us toward bordering concerns. For example, various writers have demonstrated the important relationship between poverty and mental health. Some[6] go so far as to assert the total interrelatedness between these two systems: ". . . thus as a major technique against poverty the use of indigenous persons has become a major strategy for mental health"[7]. Certainly the employment of new workers previously excluded from the field of mental health extends opportunities; individuals sheared away from the ranks of the unemployed are greatly helped—but will this eradicate poverty? It is my view that we will eradicate poverty in America when enough people decide that it is an intolerable human condition. This is a matter of politics and public policy, not just a matter of psychology and mental health—though it is indisputable that survival and mental health are connected. However, by extending the concept of mental health to cover all aspects of life we make the concept meaningless. Further, by embracing all aspects of human life we run the risk of retarding the development of other forms of social action. Bayard L. Rustin, in discussing strategies for opposing racism, comments:

"If we are to have any hope of accomplishing this task, it is essential that we make important distinctions between issues of politics and problems in psychology. We should see this as a distinction between what we do in order to influence the political and economic relations in this society and what, in a more personal way, we do to achieve self knowledge and identity. Now I do not think that these are hard and fast categories that totally exclude one another. A just society certainly encourages a healthy psychology, and individuals can find personal fulfillment through political involvement. But I think we must make this distinction because in periods of great social upheaval—and we are living through such a period —there is a tendency to politicize all things including scholarship, art, friendship, and love. The most extreme form of this total politicization is totalitarianism, a stage we have not yet reached. But even a moderate form of it can be dangerous since it can lead to a politics so preoccupied with psychological issues that the goals of political action are obscured and even rendered unobtainable."[8]

How can we guard against rigidly compartmentalized thinking while simultaneously restraining powerful impulses to commit decency without discipline? There are no easy answers. Wallerstein and Smelser, in a powerfully reasoned consideration of the relationship between psychoanalysis and sociology, acknowledge that no adequate psychological theory can exist without its being at the same time social, biological, and cultural. Nevertheless they note: ". . . man's intellectual reach to this point has been too limited to create manageable theories that simultaneously encompass the panoply of interacting forces in the empirical world. Man has been caught in a dilemma; where he would try to be realistic in his understanding of the world, he has been overwhelmed by its complexities; where he simplified its complexity, he has perforce been unrealistic. He has steered his way through this dilemma historically by creating specialized and narrowed conceptual frameworks for understanding and explaining limited aspects of reality—however, this valuable and even necessary solution has also created a number of new dilemmas and dangers"[9]. The dangers they refer to are oversimplification and a reductionism that insists upon the theories of one discipline as a "nothing but" explanation of reality.

We have historical precedents for judging the dangers of unbounded mental health zeal. An example is the Juvenile Court System. Activated by a spirit of reform,

the Juvenile Court offered mental health and rehabilitation in place of justice. Only now, many years later, have
we begun to return to some of the legal safeguards that
had been stripped away.

Or consider indeterminate jail sentences: Influenced
by persuasive mental health and other reformers, California organized a system to replace punishment with
evaluation as a prelude to individualized rehabilitation.
Nonprofessionals, under the direction of mental health
consultants, widely utilize group therapy to support
these aims. We have no evidence that these services
performed on captive inmates have been of great benefit.
But we do know that prisoners in California serve six to
eight months longer for their offenses than inmates of
other states. Inmates consider the practice of indeterminate sentences anathema: "It leaves you feeling like
you're grasping at cobwebs"[10].

DILEMMAS IN PRACTICE AND TRAINING

Programs reporting the use of nonprofessionals indicate that they are employed in a wide variety of tasks.
Many thoughtful mental health writers attest to their
usefulness in providing concrete help, imaginatively
reducing external pressures, resourcefully navigating bureaucratic systems, developing self-help programs, and
establishing bridges between reticent and mistrustful
patients and mental health agencies. Others report significant community organization, recruitment, and
follow-up. Let me acknowledge at once that these tasks
are vital, especially for previously unserved groups.
Moreover, professionals have failed to provide some of
these services systematically.

Where, then, are the problems? They rise from many
sources. The first of these hinges on the direct counseling
services provided by nonprofessionals and the shift
away from this work by professionals. "Perhaps the
greatest implication for the professional is to set for
himself a new role model as planner, administrator,
supervisor, teacher, evaluator, consultant, change agent,
etc.—rather than as the one-to-one practitioner. If the pro-

fessional can see himself in these more complicated and responsible roles, he will not be threatened by what some feel is the 'take-over' of his one-to-one responsibilities by new workers. Rather, he will see his role as the very responsible one of helping and assuring that the new workers succeed in their work. This will be difficult for many professionals who have had no training for these new roles, but it is a key consideration in the use of new levels of manpower"[11].

Such a plan would certainly swell manpower ranks but with the hazard of each of these groups doing what they know least how to do. It is one thing to assert that non-professionals may be able to perform different or simpler tasks than professionals or that there are not enough professionals to do the work in any case, so that some help is better than none—although there are complicated and debatable issues in each assertion. It is another thing to imply that the work to be done is simple and easily mastered.

From what does this kind of thinking derive? In part, it rests on the view that the cause as well as "the cure" for psychological difficulty lies in the social environment. It would follow that careful individual work is less important than social action and that serious and protracted study about intrapsychic processes and how these can be changed are largely irrelevant. The problem is basically elsewhere, in the society, external to the human being. For example, "While individual behavior is important, it is less important than group behavior in attempting to unravel the social process of change. Understanding individual Black Panther members or the individual hippie lends relatively little understanding to the growth process of the Black Panther Party or the evolving process of the peace and freedom movement"[12].

These may be laudable aims, but are they mental health? In our reawakened concern for social considerations and action some would "don the mantle of healer of all social ills"[13], while assigning to the untrained the "less complicated and responsible" task of counseling the troubled.

But are these truly simple and less responsible tasks? Kubie speaks eloquently of the necessity for the slow seasoning and maturing of the clinician who must strive to achieve that "elusive but essential combination of empathy and objectivity which alone can enable us to identify with sickness as well as with health"[14].

I do not deny that there are those rare naturals who bring great giftedness to clinical work. Nor do I suggest that the training we have devised for professionals is invariably excellent. But this does not vitiate the need to know or to develop craft. There is an increasing rise in impatience about process and a pervasive anti-intellectualism that seems to value spontaneity at the expense of knowledge. Young people, disenchanted with a scientism that had grown rigorous without relevance, clamor for a different kind of knowing—through the senses, "experience," and "feeling." Intellect is suspect. The elevation of intellectuality without emotion created its own sterility. Are we now in danger of creating a new form of isolation, opening the way to theoretical nihilism and empiricism without benefit of guiding principle or concept? The pragmatic impulse in the American temperament "finds it hard ... to believe that there is such a thing as a truth that cannot be made useful"[15]—immediately. This leads to bandwagon solutions, constant and untested improvisation, and denigration of craft. Surely there are other ways of training than through our traditionally credentialed mental health programs. Perhaps challenge will result in more systematic and judicious pruning. Perhaps the questioning process will yet create a better way of inducting new workers—professionals as well as nonprofessionals—into the field of mental health. There is, however, no evidence to my knowledge that the current training of nonprofessionals is either extensive or systematic; much of it appears to be brief and hit-or-miss. In a study undertaken in the metropolitan New York area, training of paraprofessionals was described as "limited, fragmented and inadequate for the complexities of the work they must perform"[16].

Jacobson, et al. report their not so typical training

program for nonprofessionals at the Lincoln Hospital
Community Mental Health Center in which six weeks of
training precedes on-the-job training and supervision.
They appear to be encouraged by their design and the
subsequent work of their trainees. "The pre-service
training must be concerned not only with the imparting
of skills but also with the discovery, exploration, and
modification of attitudes that might impair their
learning and job functioning. The aim of the training is
three-fold: to begin to develop the knowledge and skills
necessary to the community mental health worker; to
clarify service; and to develop, modify or change specific
attitudes or feelings"[17]. Although they grant that these
objectives can only be initiated in the pre-service period
and must be carried further on the job, is this a
reasonable expectation? These workers candidly acknowledge considerable problems. They recognize that
"initially the trainees are generally ingratiating, but this
attitude is soon replaced by covert resistance and
outright flaunting of authority." We have all heard of the
explosion at Lincoln Community Mental Health Center.
Is it possible that some of it developed in response to conflicts of loyalty brought on by attempts to serve agency
and community simultaneously—two masters who are
sometimes at odds. However, tensions may develop from
a covert sense of inadequacy on the part of nonprofessional workers when they are asked to meet complex
and demanding problems with little training. But even
more, perhaps, it partly grows from a recognition that a
subtle form of paternalism was at work at Lincoln (a
paternalism not unique to that center): ". . . residents of a
disadvantaged community enter the institutional system
in a variety of roles as patients, clients, or neighbors. . . .
Under the umbrella of training it is possible to bring
about alterations in social and psychological functioning that encourages effective coping behavior rather
than decompensation in persons who might otherwise be
forced back to one or the other more dependent roles.
Such psychological alterations have a good deal in
common with those that occur in psychotherapy"[18]. If we
intend our training programs as primarily or even

largely self-help projects, as some writers advocate, do we not unwittingly confuse and demean the trainees by not frankly acknowledging this? People who assume they have come to work may not always appreciate being rescued.

Lowenkopf and Zwerling report several cases in which family health workers function as team members. Although they confirm the value of nonprofessionals in mental health programs, they raise an important question. "In addition to being members of a medical team, the family health workers also live in the community and share its attitudes. They show a great tolerance for behavioral disturbance that does not touch them personally and a reluctance to admit that their community has a wide prevalence of psychiatric disorder. Although they often have a marked degree of personal sympathy and understanding for their patients they see them as friends and neighbors and often, for example, take incomplete histories for fear of losing potential friends or of being accused of prying. *Here it seems that the price of greater intimacy is the loss of objectivity*"[19] (my emphasis). The issue of objectivity is a tantalizing one. Like intellect and professionalism it has become suspect, equated with coldness, distance, and a lack of compassion. What is objectivity? Is it not a firm respect for the evidence, a dedicated willingness to test hypotheses with some rigor? All of us defend against human suffering in a multitude of ways. To find one's own ground, neither retreating nor over-compensating, takes time and seasoning, as well as compassion and empathy. It takes patience to tolerate another's painstaking steps towards change. But more, it takes a kind of professional objectivity to permit solutions different from one's own style of problem-solving.

"A telling criticism of many nonprofessionals is that they have manifested negative feelings toward the poor. Although it is sometimes assumed that proximity to slum life automatically endows neighborhood workers with empathy and understanding, many persons who have lived in poverty share the prevailing middle class attitudes towards the poor, they tend to look down on deprived persons and tend to be contemptuous of persons who manage less well than they in what they regard as comparable circumstances. The lower classes are, as a number of studies have shown, less liberal as a group than the upper classes. And those who have themselves been the victims of social inequities may nonetheless feel that an individual is responsible for his own circumstances and those who receive aid have no right to be critical of services for which they do not pay. Fortunately such attitudes seem to be less damaging to worker-client relationships than might be anticipated"[20]. Are we certain that such attitudes are less damaging than might be anticipated?

There are other problems. "Life experience of patients and staff from the ghetto may lead to scars as well as strengths, evidenced at times in staff by a facade of indifference, hostility, and dependency or by absenteeism and 'beating the system.' In addition there are the realities of disruptive home life, frequent needs to attend to personal business during working hours, problems with child care, and personal bouts with alcoholism, family conflict and financial stress"[21].

It has been suggested that nonprofessionals bring special and superior qualities to their counseling work—enthusiasm, optimism, lack of interfering jargon, spontaneity, and great commitment. Those of us who have inducted new workers into mental health and particularly to psychotherapeutic endeavors have observed some of these positive qualities. Are we forced then to conclude that training is useless and that the untrained are invariably better able to help? While enthusiasm and spontaneity on occasion do indeed undergo change they are often replaced by experience and objectivity. It is useful to acquire some recognition that "relationship" does not invariably lead to problem-solving, and that there are limits to our capacity to help. In meeting with patients, we not only encounter another's pain and suffering, but ourselves. This is a sobering and painful process. It takes its toll on unbridled optimism.

I do not suggest that untrained or rapidly trained workers bring nothing of importance. I have already indicated that some needed services are rarely provided by some professionals. Indigenous nonprofessionals have broadened our understanding about the poor. Another gain has been the influx of minority workers. But these gains are not unmixed blessings—they carry the dangers of rhetoric and sloganeering. To be sure, this rhetoric is born of political necessity and reality but it is extended beyond the domain of politics: "Respond to the Community's mandate," as though indeed the Community is a monolithic, single-minded, clearly articulated, and thoroughly represented entity.

I am reminded of a recent social gathering during which the conversation focused on the new roles performed by mental health workers. "Change agent," "catchment area," "altering the welfare bureaucracy," "supporting the community's effort to determine its own destiny," peppered the talk. An able local politician who had remained silent caught the group's attention with his question: "What constituency elected you people to political leadership?"

It has been charged that "the mental health professional working in the inner city is putting Band-Aids on cancer if he treats only the intrapsychic phenomenon of symptoms . . . We must eliminate the causes of despair, apathy, and rebellion, revolution or riot"[22]. Are these the only two alternatives? More, do mental health professionals have the power or the tools to eliminate "despair, apathy and hopelessness," even in concert with the inner city residents who now participate in mental health actively, not simply as recipients? While professionals have an obligation to vigorously report their knowledge about the impact upon personality of damaging social conditions, they have neither the power nor the right to determine public policy.

We are also faced with the danger of succumbing to sloganeering in our highly appropriate efforts to combat racism. Until recently we paid too little attention to the deep psychic wounds inflicted by racism. We have all begun to learn that past prized color-blind attitudes held to represent a true regard for the individual were neither totally possible, realistic, or useful. Ethnic origins and specific lifestyle are proper concerns in clinical work, direct services, and therapeutic programming. Without pressure to acknowledge this and take it more deeply into account such considerations might still lie dormant. Yet, here too hyperbole can lead to distortion. While non-minority workers must overcome their ignorance about, fear of, and resistance to other cultures, minority workers must resist "the deadly and hypnotic temptation to interpret the world and all its devices in terms of race"[23]. Kaplan, et al. comment on distortions arising from such over-identification: "This is not unique to the community mental health worker; it is a common problem for all individuals who work with the mentally ill. However, special difficulties may be anticipated for staff members who were recruited in part because of social and ethnic similarities to the patient population. While these similarities tend to promote positive identification, negative reaction from their consequences can be anticipated as the other side of the coin"[24]. These writers recommend supervision to offset such reactions. Distortions arising from over-identification or insufficient knowledge cannot always be balanced by even the most adequate supervision. One cannot report what one does not see or defends against acknowledging.

The following may serve to illustrate: A local school concerned about one of its students sought help from a community health worker in referring the child for psychiatric treatment. The family received their medical care from a comprehensive health service provided by a community hospital which also housed a department of psychiatry. Psychiatric staff were invited to attend a meeting to discuss the mother's resistance. Some years earlier they had treated an older child and the mother. The mother dropped in informally to see her former worker to report that this son was doing well. It was difficult to discern what might now account for the mother's reluctance, inhospitality, and thinly veiled hostility during the community worker's home visit. As the meeting broke up, the community worker remarked that the mother was "certainly hostile, telling me she could have had my job." It was then inadvertently learned that this mother had unsuccessfully applied for a position as a community health worker herself. Of course, professionally trained workers have blind spots, yet it is in the process of training over time that one strives to eradicate or minimize these.

ROLE DELINEATION

It has been suggested that we can expand manpower resources while insuring quality mental health care by a careful delineation of roles and focal training for these. Parenthetically, it should be noted that while manpower shortages in mental health continue to be real, trained social workers and rehabilitation counselors are currently having difficulty finding jobs. I understand this problem is spreading to other mental health professions.

Aside from the real and now more often expressed irritation by nonprofessionals who view such sorting as leading to menial assignments, is it possible to tease out simpler tasks in direct work with clients and patients? This is a beguiling prospect—but one not always easily accomplished. Human beings come in different sizes, styles, and unique presentations. It is difficult to clearly assign the aims and goals of treatment even after the most extensive diagnostic process. As the work proceeds we realign our goals and strategies repeatedly, learning from the patient, our central teacher. How can we sort out simpler from more complicated patients? Is it the psychotic who needs support and reality help? Is it the neurotic with a particular symptom which we can allay readily through sympathetic listening? Or is it the poor who will now receive services from people more intimately connected with their own culture and their own life style? Are we erecting a double standard of service? The poor will again receive the least skilled services while those who can afford it will seek the expert help for which they are prepared to pay.

In the 40's an attempt was made to assign simpler tasks to social workers who were told by their psychiatric colleagues that they could do most useful work provided they did not tamper with unconscious material or the transference. Unfortunately, patients were not given similar advice. It soon became clear that social workers needed to define the limits and possibilities of their own profession, provided they shared with other mental health professionals a knowledge about the dynamics of psychological function and the treatment of individuals and small groups. It can be argued that this historical parallel strengthens the case for role diffusion since it served to augment the manpower pool. Perhaps so. However, it must be stressed that social workers offering clinical casework expected to train conceptually as well as experientially in order to develop competence and skill.

It is important to recognize that there are many ways to help people and that they are, by no means, all psychological. Helping someone find a job, a house, and a doctor are vital services, but they are not necessarily mental health activities, even if they do have mental health by-product value. The case for a network of comprehensive services is indisputable. Mental health services must be closely connected to legal, social, and medical resources to maximize their benefit. Yet even those who would delineate the roles for nonprofessionals and attempt to distinguish between psychotherapy and other tasks speak of community workers' "diminishing pathological interaction between family members," "facilitating the development of a therapeutic alliance," "providing corrective emotional experience," "undoing a patient's narcissistic regression"[25]. These comments attest to the problems in teasing out limited roles. Is there a natural drift against which we must guard if we are intent on differentiating what can be appropriately turned over to community workers?

There is certainly avowed nonprofessional resistance to performing more simple delineated tasks; but are all community workers really asking to do full direct service? Experience with one crisis service suggests that community workers and technicians are not certain they wish to be left with the total responsibility or with unclear assignments. Clearer written job descriptions were often requested; others offered many reasons for their wish to accompany professional workers in interviews at home or in the office, while others complained of insufficient training and supervision.

Role diffusion surfaces still another difficulty. Child guidance clinics used a team approach for many years in their work. For various reasons, not least of which was its lack of economy and difficulties in collaboration, the team concept yielded considerably. The team is again in vogue—but much expanded. Today the team may include the psychiatrist, psychologist, social worker, physician, learning specialist, speech or occupational therapist, lawyer, school counselor, and community workers. Obviously, no one can object to the use of necessary multiple skills. But if my recent experiences can be used as index, I have repeatedly come upon exhaustive and often exhausting reports of what might be called "psychological multi-phasics." Little attempt has been made to integrate the findings of various workers. This represents fragmented care of a new variety. When efforts are made to synthesize varied perspectives, the time spent in collaboration is extensive and costly. Recently, I had occasion to consult with a pediatric group who reported the case of a mother who became increasingly hostile and uncooperative during her child's hospitalization. Many factors accounted for the mother's distrust but her insistence upon talking only to the pediatrician rested, in part, on disorientation created by the numbers of people who expressed concern and interest in her and her child—a concern not altogether reasonable nor clear to her. Not only the workers in our field experience diffusion—some of our patients are confused, as well.

Professionals and nonprofessionals alike find ways of countering the ambiguity and anxiety created by diffusion. In one center, in which each staff member—professional, clerical, or student—was given an equal vote in developing policy and administrative structure with the expressed aim of "breaking down the traditional separation of the mental health disciplines" a "shadow" parallel community mental health organization was discovered within the "official" organization[26]. Is it necessary to abrogate leadership or destroy all hierarchial structure to properly correct for rigid authoritarianism?

The issue of role diffusion relates as much to the professional as to the non-professional. Professionals are under great pressure to reduce their psychotherapeutic work in favor of other functions. The human condition being what it is, if status and other rewards are to be found in work other than direct service, there will be a natural drift in such directions. Application for extensive clinical training will diminish; programs offering such training will also diminish. Who then, even among the supervisors of community mental health services, will be well trained in clinical skills? Who will provide the corrective clinical supervision needed by nonprofessionals? Elsewhere I have described a program designed without sufficient knowledge of the dynamics of human functioning which created for its young clients as many problems as it solved[27].

If professional mental health workers trained in clinical work are continually pressured to do things they are less well trained to do, will we not eventually create a vacuum of expert clinicians? Absurd? Not quite. We have witnessed an increasing tendency in many social work schools to teach *about* casework, rather than to teach it directly. As the doctorate becomes a requirement for teaching, teachers with scant practice experience discuss values, competing theories, and research studies with less and less attention to direct clinical experience. While this does not account entirely for a reduced interest in casework, neither can it be altogether discounted. Like a self-fulfilling prophecy, teachers uncommitted to clinical work produce students uninterested in clinical practice. Thus practice loses value, irrespective of its merit.

There are some unusual teachers who do not require enrichment from ongoing clinical practice. But many who fail to refresh their concepts with live human encounters soon become sterile, whether they teach in schools or on the job. Thus we may increasingly have for teachers those with brief experience with patients and as time passes experiences that grow older and staler. A foreign visitor to this country, commenting on what he considered a strange American custom, noted that "they take a young man who has shown great promise in some field and promote him to a higher position in which it is impossible for him to continue doing that for which he has shown such promise"[28]. We seem bent on enshrining the Peter Principle.

CONSULTATION: DILEMMAS AND PROBLEMS

The hope we have riding on consultation to nonprofessionals obscures some of its problems. The use of nonprofessional workers relies heavily on consultation for insuring the nonprofessional's effectiveness. Lowenkopf and Zwerling report an illustration of a community worker who masked her wish for magical solutions from her consultant. Her need to solve complicated and unresolvable family problems served as a measure not only of her competence but of her continued status in the community.

A consultant's failure to solve the unsolvable creates frustration and antagonism. Indigenous workers, reluctant to acknowledge emotional pathology often experience the consultant as disappointing or withholding when he cannot provide answers in terms they find acceptable. Should the consultant persist in his psychological stance, the consultee may become frustrated and even overtly hostile. When we do not share some similar body of knowledge, there is no common frame of reference. The shared concern for the patient may be insufficient to outweigh misunderstandings, differences in goal and appreciation for the limits of helping. Repeated experiences over time may reduce such difficulty. Other times the difficulties are displaced upon patients or the institution. Energy is drawn away from the work as the staff splinters into opposing and hostile groups. Pushed by worker's demands for solutions, intent on being useful, eager to avoid open hostility and conflict, aware that psychological explanations may affront, fearful of facing the charge of racism when minority workers are involved, consultants often experience considerable confusion, frustration, and just plain misery. Some compromise their consultations and water down their observations and suggestions. Others who cannot lick them join them to become social reformers, though they may have scant knowledge in reforming. Others stand and persist in their work. In one project with which I am familiar three of four psychiatric consultants left their posts within a year and a half. (I am told that this is not an isolated instance.) The remaining consultant regularly sought out colleagues in another setting for repeated and informal consultations in order to assure some distance and objectivity.

With all due respect to admired colleagues who have worked in the field of consultation, its theory is still in infancy. Despite a growing body of literature, much of consultation theory originated in settings other than those which deal with impoverished populations. There is considerable confusion for consultants today as they try to apply what is known of consultation to this new group. I do not contend that consultation cannot profitably spread mental health services, but there are limits to its effectiveness. Culling from my own experience, teachers repeatedly ask for direct services within the schools. Many would gladly exchange such help for the consultation they receive, affirming that they cannot do the job for which they themselves were trained while confronted by the many children who for emotional reasons cannot learn. This, despite the fact that consultation had on occasion helped to produce positive teacher-initiated changes within the school.

CONCLUSIONS AND SUMMARY

Concerns about role diffusion rest on new and emerging trends in community mental health. These in turn have been sharply influenced by rapidly changing values in the general culture. Traditional practice, delivery of services, the value of training, previously valued concepts of professionalism, objectivity and intellectuality are all open to question. The role of community workers in direct service and as change agents places considerable strain upon their resources. No less stressful are the confusions and doubts confronting the professional as he struggles to maintain, extend, or clarify his role. The shift and drift in function, sometimes designed and sometimes by default, presses toward role diffusion.

This adds to further questioning, dispute, and confrontation. The difficulty in determining the boundaries of mental health goals and efforts further complicates an already complicated problem.

The realities are difficult ones and cannot always wait for neat and clear responses. Manpower problems are real and insistent; we may not be permitted the luxury of slowly testing whether role diffusion creates more problems than it resolves. Yet we are often tempted to make virtues of necessities.

Despite a highly sophisticated material technology we do not yet have an adequate technology to determine how best to help human beings in psychological trouble. As surely as "life is with people" we can be certain that untrained people have always helped others and can do so now. The question is how best to utilize natural talent and build upon it, how to define tasks commensurate with talents and skill? We must face the potential hazards, problems, and dilemmas and use our understanding to chart a course for action. We cannot allow an awareness of the exigencies to draw us willy nilly into intemperate action.

Despite the confusion and turbulence we can already count some important gains brought by the new thinking in community mental health: A heightened concern for and sensitivity to the disadvantaged, a willingness to be more attentive to social and cultural forces, a reduction of professional insularity and authoritarian attitudes and systems, a concern for developing a network of services closer geographically and psychologically to the lives of people in trouble, a wish to reach the previously unserved, and the willingness to consider prevention as well as remediation.

And the possible costs? Omnipotent over-promise; subtle paternalism rather than effective partnership; a double-track system of help, one for the poor, another for the middle and affluent class; a yielding to pressure rather than action through conviction; solutions by experts or alleged experts to problems which properly belong to the total citizenry; sloganeering in place of reason; a "retreat from patients" to less well known but more currently esteemed endeavors; the hazard of creating a vacuum of skilled clinicians; a willingness to settle for partial truths and the "fluctuating extremes of fashionable opinion"; romanticizing impoverishment; the confusion of ideas with their abuses and the risk, then, of turning from the task of repair.

The past decade is not alone in its turbulence. There was a

> "great wave of enthusiasm for wholesale measures of reform . . . that wave brought with it many changes that made better social casework possible, but some of the leading social worker reformers of the period lost their heads to this extent . . . they were sure that legislation and propaganda, between them, would render social work with and for individuals quite unnecessary, and they did not hesitate to say so . . . during all that period, I know, it was uphill work to interest either the public or the social reformers in any reform that dealt with people one by one instead of in great masses. It was a time of slogans. Do not misunderstand me. I am as eager to see poverty eradicated as anyone can be but the verb 'to abolish' has for its synonym 'to repeal, to revoke, to rescind, to recall, to abrogate, to annul', and I submit that poverty is not a political or even a social status to be abolished or rescinded by an amendment to the constitution of the United States or by a Presidential proclamation . . . prevention is another one of those words, which as used in proverb and slogan, has been much abused. Who that is familiar, for instance, with the history of the tuberculosis campaign s in this country can ever place 'prevention' and 'cure' in antithesis to each other again? The two processes interplay at each turn, and cure, in and of itself, is a form of prevention, for we learn how to prevent by honestly trying to cure. In other words, prevention is one of the end results of a series of processes which include research, individual treatment, public education, legislation and then (by retraced steps) back to the administrative adaptations which make the intent of legislation real again in the individual case.
>
> The interplay of these wholesale and retail processes is an indispensable factor in any social progress which is to be permanent."[30]

These words were retrospectively written in 1924 about the period between 1905 and 1914 by Mary Richmond, the founder of professional social work. We are in such a time as Mary Richmond describes years ago. How much have we learned in the intervening years?

We have need for revolutionaries—those who challenge and reject tradition—and evolutionaries—those who would salvage and link older views to newer concepts. But perhaps we need even more those who recognize that every new trial and advance creates new and difficult problems which require more than good will for their solution.

REFERENCES

1. Seymour R. Kaplan, Levon Z. Boyajian, & Betty Meltzer, The Role of the Non-Professional Worker. From Henry Grunebaum: *The Practice of Community Mental Health,* Little, Brown & Co., 1970, p. 596.

2. Robin Huws Jones, Social Values and Social Work Education, *Social Values in an Age of Discontent,* ed. Kathcrine Kendell, Council on Social Work Education, 1970, p. 35.

3. A. W. Whitehead as quoted in Robert White, *Lives and Progress,* 2nd Edition, New York, Holt, Reinhart & Winston, 1966, p. 1.

4. Charles Frankel, Social Values and Professional Values, *Journal of Education for Social Work,* Council of Social Work Education, Spring, 1969, p. 32.

5. Ibid.

6. Leonard J. Duhl, What Mental Health Services are Needed for the Poor, *Poverty and Mental Health,* ed. Milton Greenblatt, Paul Emery, Bernard Geneck, Jr. Psychiatric Research Report, American Psychiatric Assoc., January, 1967, pp. 72-78.

7. Seymour R. Kaplan, Levon Z. Boyajian, & Betty Meltzer, The Role of the Non-Professional Worker. From Henry Grunebaum: *The Practice of Community Mental Health,* Little, Brown & Co., 1970, p. 595.

8. Bayard Rustin, A Word to Black Students, *Dissent,* Nov-Dec 1970, p. 583.

9. Robert S. Wallerstein and Neil Smelser, Psychoanalysis and Sociology: Articulations and Applications. *Int'l. J. Psychoanalysis,* #50, 1969, p. 694.

10. As reported in San Francisco Chronicle, 10 March 1971.

11. Roles and Functions for Different Levels of Mental Health Workers—A report of a symposium on Manpower Utilization for Mental Health, Dec., 1969, p. 68. Community College Mental Health Worker Project, Southern Regional Educational Board, 130 Sixth Street, N.W., Atlanta, Georgia.

12. Douglas L. Foster, Change in the Black Community: Revolution or Evolution. *American J. of Orthopsychiatry,* 41:2, March 1971, p. 227. Digests of Papers—48th Annual Meeting, American Orthopsychiatric Association, Washington, D.C. March 21-24, 1971.

13. Ira M. Steisel, Issues in Delivery of Child Psychological Care by Paraprofessionals. Presented at American Association of Psychiatric Services for Children, November 6, 1970.
14. Lawrence S. Kubie, Retreat from Patients. *Archives of General Psychiatry* Vol. 24, Feb. 1971, p. 99.
15. Richard Hofstadter, The Importance of Comity in American History, *Columbia Forum*, Vol. XIII, Winter 1970, No. 4.
16. Harry Gottesfeld, Chongik Rhee, Glenn Parker, A Study of the Role of Paraprofessionals in Community Mental Health. *Community Mental Health Journal*, Vol. 6 (4), 1970, p. 288.
17. Sally L. Jacobson, Melvin Roman, & Seymour R. Kaplan, Training Non-Professional Workers. *The Practice of Community Mental Health*, ed. Henry Grunebaum, Little, Brown & Co., 1970, pp. 625-645.
18. Jacobson, et al., p. 641.
19. Eugene Lowenkopf & Israel Zwerling, Psychiatric Services in a Neighborhood Health Center. *American J. Psychiatry*, 127:7, Jan. 1971, p. 919.
20. Gertrude S. Goldberg, *Non-Professionals in the Human Services*, ed. Chas. Grosser, Wm. E. Henry, James G. Kelly, Jossey Bass, Inc., San Francisco 1969, p. 23.
21. June Jackson Christmas, Hilda Wallace, & Jose Edwards, New Careers and Mental Health Services: Fantasy or Future. *American J. Psychiatry*, 126:10, April 1970. pp. 132-3.
22. Hiawatha Harris, Health Self-Determination. *American J. Psychiatry*, 126:10, April 1970, p. 126.
23. Ralph Ellison as quoted in Bayard Rustin, A Word to Black Youth, *Dissent*, Nov-Dec 1970, p. 584.
24. Kaplan, et al., op. cit. p. 604.
25. Kaplan, et al., op. cit.
26. Allen J. Enelow & W. Donald Weston, Jr., Cooperation or Chaos: The Mental Health Administrator's Dilemma. *American J. Orthopsychiatry*, 41:2, March 1971 p. 288. Digests of Papers—48th Annual Meeting, American Orthopsychiatric Association, Washington, D.C., March 21-24, 1971.
27. Shirley Cooper, The Swing to Community Mental Health, *Social Casework*, May 1968.
28. Lawrence S. Kubie, op. cit. p. 104.
29. Lowenkopf, et al., op. cit.
30. The Long View, Russell Sage Foundation, 1930. pp. 586-587.

The Research Study

THE RESEARCH STUDY

The research on issues in community mental health started with a literature search covering 1967, 1968, and 1969, the years preceding the data collection and analysis itself. Every article and book that could be found through review and indexing services that purported to be related to community mental health was read and every general statement relating to the author's philosophy or view about community mental health was extracted. Examples of statements follow: "A community mental health center should treat everyone, regardless of their age, psychiatric diagnosis or degree of disturbance." "The same clinical team should be responsible for each patient's initial evaluation, treatment and followup." "Community mental health programs are committed to political positions rather than health concerns." "Mass treatment or mass prevention methods in psychiatry will only lead to disappointments." "White professionals are not able to work successfully with black clients." "Successful treatment of mental illness requires treatment of society as a whole." "A community mental health center should be hospital centered." "The establishment of community mental health centers will result in ordinary problems of living being interpreted as psychiatric problems." The numerous statements that were culled from articles and books were examined for duplications of meaning and the duplications were eliminated. What remained then were more than four hundred statements. Since these were too many statements for respondents' reactions to the questionnaire form that was contemplated, one hundred statements were chosen randomly. Some of the positive statements were changed and phrased negatively to minimize the effect of response sets. The statements were put into a questionnaire form in which the respondent could rate each statement on a six-point scale ranging from "strongly agree" to "strongly disagree" according to his beliefs. The respondent did not give his name to assure anonymity and probably more frank answers, but was asked for some background information such as age, sex, occupation, etc.

The questionnaire was pretested to determine the clarity of items and instructions. The wording of items and instructions was modified accordingly in the final questionnaire.

All agencies in the New York metropolitan area known to have a community mental health program were asked to participate in the study and asked to administer the questionnaire to their staffs. Almost all agreed to do so on the basis that it would be voluntary for each staff person. Eighteen agencies cooperated and 830 staff members completed questionnaires. These included psychiatric nurses, psychiatrists, psychologists, social workers, and mental health paraprofessionals. The staff involved both those in the community mental health programs as well as those in other mental health units of the facility, since sharp distinctions between those who were in the community mental health program and those who were in conventional psychiatric programs were often difficult to establish. The average percentage of staff of institutions that responded to the questionnaire was 50% with a range of 20% to 81%.

The questionnaire data was subjected to a principal components factor analysis and rotation was by normal varimax. Six factors evolved.* Items were listed under the factor for which they had the highest loading. The factors were then named.

RESULTS

Table 1 lists the issues (factors) and the percentage of

* The decision to accept for rotation six factors was based on a sharp drop in the seventh latent root and the relatively small residual correlations following the extraction of the sixth factor.

TABLE 1
Issues and Their % of Common Variance

#	Name of Issue	% Of Common Variance
1	COMMUNITY CONTEXT	26
2	RADICALISM	17
3	TRADITIONAL PSYCHOTHERAPY	17
4	PREVENTION	14
5	EXTENDING THE DEFINITION OF MENTAL HEALTH	14
6	ROLE DIFFUSION	12
		100

common variance accounted for by each. Relatively the strongest issue is "Community Context." Stated another way, in the late 1969's the most important issue for those who wrote professionally about community mental health was "Community Context."

RELATIONSHIP OF INDEPENDENT VARIABLES TO ISSUES

Each issue (factor) was considered as a dependent variable and profession, ethnicity, age, sex, type of work, and institutional affiliation were considered as independent variables. Through cumulative multiple regression analyses the degree to which each independent variable was related to the dependent variables as well as to what degree combinations of independent variables were related to the dependent variables was determined. Through these statistical procedures the relationship of independent and dependent variables could be studied, partialling out the contaminating effects of independent variables on each other. For example, in studying the possible relationship between the sex of respondents and their ratings of a given issue, sex is not truly independent but related to professional membership; nurses and social workers tend to be female, physicians, male. Correlations between sex and a given issue really may represent differences in professional membership and the issues. The multiple regression analysis allows professional mem-

TABLE 2
Relationship (Expressed in %) of Background Variables and Issues

Issues	Background Variables						
	1 Profession	2 Ethnic Identification	3 Age	4 Sex	5 Type of Work	6 Institutional Affiliation	Total of all Variables
1. COMMUNITY CONTEXT	12	1	3	0	6	8	30
2. RADICALISM	4	1	2	1	0	4	12
3. TRADITIONAL PSYCHOTHERAPY	16	4	0	0	3	4	27
4. PREVENTION	3	1	3	0	1	3	11
5. EXTENDING THE DEFINITION OF MENTAL HEALTH	2	4	2	1	0	6	15
6. ROLE DIFFUSION	2	0	3	0	5	6	16

bership to be accounted for (or partialled out) before studying the relationship of sex as such and an issue.

In Table 2 the incremental relationship of the background (independent) variables to each of the issues is expressed in terms of percent of variance accounted for on the issue. An arbitrarily determined cutoff of 2% or more was considered worthy of note (2% is highly significant statistically) and is described in the text.

1. Community Context

There is a moderate association between membership in the different professions and "Community Context" (12% of the variance is accounted for by membership). The greatest departure from the average stand among the various professions is that of the medical profession; it is the profession most opposed to this issue. Other professions are more positively inclined, with paraprofessionals being the most positively inclined.

Ethnicity does not have any signicant relationship to this issue when adjustments have been made for professional membership. Neither does sex when adjustments for previous independent variables have been made. However, age, institutional affiliation, and whether one is primarily in community mental health do have significant relationships to the issue. Those who are primarily in community mental health and are younger are more positive on this issue.

2. Radicalism

There is a small, but statistically significant, relationship between membership in different professions and "Radicalism" (accounting for 4% of the variance). Again, as on issue 1, the medical profession is the profession most in disagreement with "Radicalism." Ethnicity, sex, and participation in community mental health work do not have any significant relationship to this issue but institutional affiliation and age do. The younger are more in favor of "Radicalism," the older less in favor, as might have been expected for this type of issue.

3. Traditional Psychotherapy

There is a moderately strong association between membership in the different professions and "Traditional Psychotherapy" (accounting for 16% of the variance). On a relative basis the social workers and psychologists are least in favor of the use of traditional psychotherapeutic methods in community mental health, physicians and nurses have intermediate positions, while paraprofessionals are most in favor of the use of traditional psychotherapeutic methods.

Age and sex do not have any significant relationship to this issue but ethnicity, community mental health work, and institutional affiliation do. Whites and those primarily in community mental health work are least in favor of traditional psychotherapy. Blacks and Puerto Ricans are more in favor of these traditional methods.

4. Prevention

There is a small but statistically significant association between membership in the different professions and "Prevention" (accounting for 3% of the variance). Relatively, paraprofessionals are most in favor of doing preventative work, psychologists most opposed. Ethnicity and sex do not have any significant relationship to this issue but institutional affiliation and age do. The below-30 age group is most in favor of prevention, the 50-and-over group least.

5. Extending the Definition of Mental Health

There is a small statistically significant association between membership in different professions and "Extending the Definition of Mental Health" (accounting for 2% of the variance). Relatively, social workers are most in favor of an extended definition of mental health. There is no significant association between type of work and sex to this issue but institutional affiliation, ethnicity, and age are significantly related. Whites and younger mental health workers believe more in "Extending the Definition of Mental Health."

6. Role Diffusion

There is a small but statistically significant association between membership in different professions and "Role Diffusion." Psychologists seem most in favor of "Role Diffusion." However, this is probably an artifact. The difference between psychologists and other professions is based mainly on one questionnaire item directly relating to psychologists: "An important role for the psychologist in the Community Mental Health Center is to develop new treatment approaches." Psychologists tend to "strongly agree" on this item while the reaction of other professions is varied. If this item had been eliminated from the questionnaire it is likely that there would have been no significant association between membership in different professions and the issue of "Role Diffusion."

There is no significant relationship between this issue and ethnicity or sex but work in community mental health programs and age are significantly related. Those who are younger mental health workers and are primarily in community mental health work believe more in "Role Diffusion."

Since institutional affiliation was significantly associated with each of the issues, the data for institutional affiliation were further examined. Seventeen institutions that participated in the study were ranked according to their staff's standing on each issue (one institution of the eighteen which originally participated was not included in the rankings because relatively few staff were involved in the study). The rankings appear in Table 3. Note that rankings on issues by institutions do not seem to follow a consistent pattern. No institution's staff could be considered relatively "liberal" on all issues. Only one institution's staff (institution #10) can be considered relatively "conservative" on all issues.

Over-all, the cumulative relationships of the background (independent) variables to the issues are moderately strong by social science standards. The background variables account for 11% to 30% of the variance of the issues (Table 2). The relatively strongest relationships exist between the background variables and the

TABLE 3
Ranking of Institutions on Staff Beliefs
About Community Mental Health Issues

Institution	Issue					
	1	2	3	4	5	6
1	6	8	12	1	10	5
2	5	14	7	7	16	4
3	9	2	5	4	4	12
4	4	6	13	14	8	3
5	16	5	8	5	7	16
6	14	13	2	2	15	14
7	11	4	9	3	3	7
8	7	15	11	15	17	10
9	2	1	17	17	9	2
10	17	17	1	1	12	15
11	12	16	6	13	6	9
12	15	11	10	6	11	13
13	13	12	16	9	1	17
14	8	7	4	8	5	11
15	10	9	3	12	2	6
16	3	10	14	10	13	1
17	1	3	15	11	14	8

Key:
    Issues: 1. Community Context
               2. Radicalism
               3. Traditional Psychotherapy
               4. Prevention
               5. Extending the Definition of Mental Health
               6. Role Diffusion
    Ranking: 1. Most Favorable Toward Issue
               17. Most Unfavorable Toward Issue

issues "Community Context" and "Traditional Psychotherapy." The weakest relationships are between the background variables and "Prevention" and "Radicalism."

DISCUSSION

This research study covers the domain of what has appeared in the literature under community mental health. The research has identified the principal dimensions or issues in the field. Community context, radicalism, traditional psychotherapy, prevention, extended mental health definitions, and expanded professional and nonprofessional roles are the crucial issues at the beginning of the 1970's. Since each of these issues has been and will continue to be a source of ideological controversy and power struggles it is worthwhile to look carefully at the description of each issue, consider its implications, and decide for ourselves if the issue is one on which we choose to take sides.

"Community Context," relatively the strongest issue, in essence makes up the first word of "community mental health." It is more frequently given lip service by community mental health organizations than carried into practice. The implications of this issue are that services function directly in the community and not at a hospital or social agency base; that the community people determine their needs and the kinds of services they want from the community mental health center rather than the mental health professional; that communication among community mental health staff be in social terminology rather than medical terminology; and that the staff itself operate as an open, democratic community. Few community mental health centers fulfill these components of "Community Context." While some services may be actually in the community, for example, storefronts or mobile mental health teams, most services of the community mental health center are likely to be institutionally based. Institutional services may be forbidding or difficult to negotiate for community people. When people in the local neighborhood make requests for specific services from the community mental health center such as help with housing or welfare, the center tends to refer them elsewhere, to other institutions. In so doing the center believes it is acting appropriately but actually may be contributing to fragmentation of services and an increase in community frustration and thus creating a poor model of mental health.

More often than not the community mental health center's staff operates on hierarchical lines rather than as a democratic, close-knit unit. Yet how the staff functions with each other is likely to have its counterparts in how the staff functions in the community. Distance between staff members will probably be reflected in distance between staff and community. One of the implications here is that the community mental health center's internal organizational philosophy may be directly related to its effectiveness in the community. Also, techniques such as sensitivity training for staff aimed at making the staff more aware of their relationships with each other and helping to overcome those impediments that keep staff members from feeling close to each other—differences in training, status, etc.—can be important for community work.

"Radicalism," with its stress on the need for rapid change in the field, political involvement, methods reaching large masses of people, and community control of the community mental health center, has become an increasingly important issue in recent years. A number of confrontations between the "establishment" and "radicals" have taken place at community mental health centers, sometimes with an aftermath of a deeply divided staff and chaotic conditions. The struggle in community mental health seems to parallel similar struggles in the welfare and educational fields. One element of this issue, the involving of local citizens in a policy-making role for the community mental health center, has federal governmental backing and the 1970's are likely to see community residents increasingly represented as board members of policy-making bodies.

"Traditional Psychotherapy," which is characterized by individual psychotherapy, long-term treatment, a psychoanalytic orientation and a private practice model, has been severely compromised in most community mental health centers by the center's need to address itself to the service demands of large masses of people. However, the issue is still very much alive and many staff people and administrators consider traditional psychotherapy the preferred method of treatment that should be applied as much as is feasible. This issue may be stronger in the New York area, where the research study was done, than in the rest of the country because of the concentration of training facilities in New York emphasizing traditional psychotherapeutic approaches.

"Prevention," with its emphasis on crisis intervention,

consultation, early identification of emotional problems, and follow-up, has been one of the major directions in which community mental health centers have moved away from traditional mental health services. Secondary and tertiary preventative programs have been more common than primary prevention programs. On the face of it, prevention would hardly seem to be a controversial issue at all, but critics have questioned its assumptions and effectiveness. There is relatively little research on prevention to supply ammunition to its advocates or critics.

An extended definition of mental health and expanded professional and nonprofessional roles seem consonant with community mental health. However, these are controversial issues, with those who take the negative side of these issues pointing out the dilemmas that arise in such areas as professional responsibility, conflicts with other professions, rights of clients, and the ethics of proceeding beyond one's skills and knowledge.

Of the many kinds of gaps that often divide people—age, sex, occupation, etc.—which contribute to differences of viewpoint on the critical issues in community mental health? Occupation, engagement in community mental health work, ethnicity, age, and institutional affiliation seem to be important variables related to people's belief systems. It is notable that those of the medical profession and those age 50 and older tend to be conservative on the community mental health issues. These groups usually have the most influential positions in mental health and what this portends for the future is a continuing power struggle in which those with the most power will be defending entrenched, conservative positions.

Mental health workers who state that their work is primarily in community mental health tend to believe more than others in community context and role diffusion and less in traditional psychotherapeutic procedures. Black and Puerto Rican mental health workers believe less in an extended definition of mental health and more in traditional psychotherapeutic procedures than do white mental health workers. Paraprofessionals also believe more in traditional psychotherapy than do other mental health workers. These groups represent the ones newest to the mental health field and it is they who are most in favor of traditional treatment forms that others in the field have begun to abandon. On this issue they represent a conservative element.

It is common to think of institutions that have community mental health programs as "radical," "liberal," "conservative," or "reactionary" in their views of community mental health. However, this study indicates that institutions generally cannot be characterized in this way. Institutions typically are conservative on some issues and liberal on others. An institution's staff may have little belief in community context, radicalism, and traditional psychotherapeutic procedures yet may strongly espouse an extended definition of mental health, prevention, and role diffusion. An institution's ideological stance in community mental health defies a simple, definitive, unidimensional statement.

In a more general sense, the critical issues in community mental health reflect the transition of traditional mental health facilities into community mental health centers. Previously a conventional mental health agency, such as a hospital psychiatric division or an outpatient clinic, tended to conduct its operation solely within its own facilities, offered few forms of treatment to a limited number of patients, and employed personnel from the established mental health disciplines to carry out these functions. When Congress established The Community Mental Health Centers Act and a number of conventional mental health facilities decided to become community mental health centers or part of such centers, they found they were faced with new mandates. The center was to serve all people from large populations in a given geographical area and offer a large variety of services including consultation and education in the community. The new mandates made the old ways of operating seem inappropriate or at least inefficient.

New approaches and ways of carrying on the business of mental health with large numbers of people in the community were suggested: having mental health facilities located throughout the community; involving community people in the planning of services; using short-term treatment modalities, group approaches and social action techniques; employing paraprofessionals and volunteers to carry out activities formerly done by professionals; emphasizing prevention. Innovations such as these met mixed receptions. In a number of instances these approaches went contrary to established, vested interests and were opposed vigorously. Many mental health administrators and professionals who might have been amenable to new services or service delivery systems that could reach large masses of people felt that some or many of the new approaches being suggested were anathema to them; such approaches seemed undesirable and/or unworkable. The research study reported in this book indicates that the younger mental health workers are more favorably inclined to the innovative approaches. Older and medically trained mental health workers are more likely to be opposed. Paraprofessionals, although strongly community oriented and favorable to preventative methods, also are advocates of traditional one-to-one, long-term treatment. Most institutions favor certain of the new approaches but are opposed to others. No clearcut pattern of "liberalism" or "conservatism" seems to emerge among an institution's staff regarding the utilization of innovative approaches.

This seems to be the state of community mental health in the early 1970's. The critical issues of today revolve around how much to hold on to established mental health methods and approaches and how much to adopt new ones. Controversy rages at all levels.

APPENDIX

ISSUES IN
COMMUNITY MENTAL HEALTH

You are being asked to participate in a study of opinions about community mental health. Your participation will supply valuable information.

On the following pages you will find a list of statements directly or indirectly related to community mental health. Please read each statement and then indicate to what extent you agree or disagree with it. You should do this by circling next to each statement the one of the six symbols which best represents your own feelings about this statement.

Please make sure that you circle a symbol for each statement. Leave none of the items blank and make only one circle for each item. Like everyone else you will feel that you do not know how to judge some of these statements. When this occurs, please make the best estimate you can. You should not spend more than a few seconds on each item. If it seems difficult to make up your mind make the best judgement you can and go on to the next item.

Please do *not* write your name. Thank you for your cooperation.

Circle AAA, if you strongly agree
Circle AA, if you moderately agree
(generally agree with some reservations)
Circle A, if you slightly agree
(more arguments for than against)
Circle D, if you slightly disagree
(more arguments against than for)
Circle DD, if you moderately disagree
(generally disagree with some reservations)
Circle DDD, if you strongly disagree

	Strongly Agree	Moderately Agree	Slightly Agree	Slightly Disagree	Moderately Disagree	Strongly Disagree	Factor	Loading
1. A community mental health center should treat everyone; regardless of their age, psychiatric diagnosis or degree of disturbance.	AAA	AA	A	D	DD	DDD	6	.20
2. The orthodox psychoanalyst is needed in community mental health work.	AAA	AA	A	D	DD	DDD	3	.34
3. A community mental health program should examine the policies and procedures of courts.	AAA	AA	A	D	DD	DDD	1	.25
4. Psychiatric patients should be employed for such tasks as making home visits to other psychiatric patients.	AAA	AA	A	D	DD	DDD	6	.45
5. The community mental health movement is moving too rapidly with insufficient planning.	AAA	AA	A	D	DD	DDD	2	-.47
6. It is better to keep an emotionally disturbed child at home even if his parents are mentally ill than to institutionalize him.	AAA	AA	A	D	DD	DDD		
7. Traditional psychotherapeutic methods are effective with low income pa-	AAA	AA	A	D	DD	DDD	6	.34

Item	AAA	AA	A	D	DD	DDD		
sponsible for each patient's initial evaluation, treatment and follow up.	AAA	AA	A	D	DD	DDD	4	.21
9. Research findings and evaluative studies are not helpful in improving practice.	AAA	AA	A	D	DD	DDD	2	-.28
10. The Community Mental Health Center should focus its efforts on general areas of community concern, such as racial tension.	AAA	AA	A	D	DD	DDD	1	.47
11. All important administrative decisions should be voted on by both staff and patients.	AAA	AA	A	D	DD	DDD	1	.59
12. Low-income persons are not sophisticated enough to participate in policy making in health agencies.	AAA	AA	A	D	DD	DDD	2	-.37
13. The terms "mental illness" and "treatment" should be replaced by "psycho-social disabilities," and "reeducation."	AAA	AA	A	D	DD	DDD	1	.45
14. Emergency services should not be manned by beginning psychiatric students.	AAA	AA	A	D	DD	DDD	6	-.18
15. Professionals and non-professionals should be trained together.	AAA	AA	A	D	DD	DDD	1	.46
16. Money would be better spent in increasing the budgets of welfare services than of mental health services.	AAA	AA	A	D	DD	DDD	1	.35

	Strongly Agree	Moderately Agree	Slightly Agree	Slightly Disagree	Moderately Disagree	Strongly Disagree	Factor	Loading
17. A social club by ex-psychiatric patients should have close professional supervision.	AAA	AA	A	D	DD	DDD	3	.28
18. It is important that a community mental health center have its own rehabilitation services even if there are other local agencies with excellent rehabilitation services.	AAA	AA	A	D	DD	DDD	3	.48
19. Social workers who serve as consultants to schools should concentrate their efforts more on the interactions of the school organization rather than on the problems of individual children.	AAA	AA	A	D	DD	DDD	3	-.32
20. The Day, Evening and Week-End Hospital will replace the Mental Hospital.	AAA	AA	A	D	DD	DDD	1	.53
21. Drug addiction is primarily a psychiatric problem.	AAA	AA	A	D	DD	DDD	3	.46
22. The Community Mental Health Center's staff should be actively involved in treatment only when the problem promises to respond to brief interven-								

making and decisions, mental health professionals are not likely to be at-tracted to community mental health.

	AAA	AA	A	D	DD	DDD		
(cont.)	AAA	AA	A	D	DD	DDD	2	-.39
24. A great risk of the Community Mental Health Center is that patients will be sent home prematurely.	AAA	AA	A	D	DD	DDD	2	-.38
25. Successful treatment of mental illness requires treatment of society as a whole.	AAA	AA	A	D	DD	DDD	1	.61
26. Community mental health resources can provide little help to the mentally retarded.	AAA	AA	A	D	DD	DDD	5	-.39
27. Non-professionals, with training, can learn to be psychotherapists as well as or better than professional therapists.	AAA	AA	A	D	DD	DDD	1	.40
28. Community mental health implies social control and allies the mental health practitioner closely with judges, police and other coercive forces.	AAA	AA	A	D	DD	DDD	5	-.29
29. The most effective way to treat the emotionally disturbed child is by long term psychotherapy of the child and his parents.	AAA	AA	A	D	DD	DDD	3	.59
30. Community mental health programs are committed to political positions rather than health concerns.	AAA	AA	A	D	DD	DDD	2	-.34

	Strongly Agree	Moderately Agree	Slightly Agree	Slightly Disagree	Moderately Disagree	Strongly Disagree	Factor	Loading
31. Police are potentially one of the most suitable groups for training in family crisis intervention.	AAA	AA	A	D	DD	DDD	6	.41
32. An important role for the social worker is to teach people how to deal with social agencies.	AAA	AA	A	D	DD	DDD	6	.37
33. Diagnostic services should involve the whole family in family evaluation sessions.	AAA	AA	A	D	DD	DDD	1	.41
34. A community mental health program should be hospital centered.	AAA	AA	A	D	DD	DDD	1	-.35
35. It is not necessary for a mental health consultant to a social agency to have a detailed knowledge of the agency's policies and procedures.	AAA	AA	A	D	DD	DDD	5	-.34
36. The Community Mental Health Center should be involved in such tasks as organizing block associations, tenant councils, and welfare client organizations.	AAA	AA	A	D	DD	DDD	1	.54

	AAA	AA	A	D	DD	DDD		
37. Most schizophrenic patients need hospitalization and should not be kept with their families.	AAA	AA	A	D	DD	DDD	3	.36
38. Socio-economic factors are highly related to mental illness.	AAA	AA	A	D	DD	DDD	1	.31
39. Using psychiatric manpower mainly for "consultation" results in responsibility that is professionally fragmented.	AAA	AA	A	D	DD	DDD	6	-.23
40. Bartenders, police officers, clergymen and other "gatekeepers" have a more crucial role in community mental health than the community mental health professionals.	AAA	AA	A	D	DD	DDD	1	.33
41. When a psychiatric nurse recognizes that a child is being psychologically damaged she should be able to compel the parents to begin a treatment program.	AAA	AA	A	D	DD	DDD	3	.45
42. The private practice model in which the patient is free to choose his own therapist, responsibility is concentrated in one therapist and the therapist is an agent of the patient, should be followed as much as possible in a community mental health center.	AAA	AA	A	D	DD	DDD	3	.36

	Strongly Agree	Moderately Agree	Slightly Agree	Slightly Disagree	Moderately Disagree	Strongly Disagree	Factor	Loading
43. Mental problems of the lower socio-economic groups are so intertwined with real social problems that they rarely can be solved by the skills of the psychiatrist.	AAA	AA	A	D	DD	DDD	1	.41
44. A walk in (emergency) psychiatric clinic should serve patients who do not present psychiatric emergencies.	AAA	AA	A	D	DD	DDD	6	.34
45. Preventative psychiatry should concentrate on strengthening the family unit.	AAA	AA	A	D	DD	DDD	4	.53
46. When a community mental health center and a welfare agency collaborate, staff is utilized most effectively if the center's mental health personnel serve as consultants to the welfare agency's workers.	AAA	AA	A	D	DD	DDD	4	.50
47. Volunteers should be encouraged to establish personal relationships with psychiatric patients.	AAA	AA	A	D	DD	DDD	6	.45

	AAA	AA	A	D	DD	DDD		
48. A community mental health center should not have facilities for long term care of the aged.	AAA	AA	A	D	DD	DDD	6	-.22
49. The private practitioner should continue to have responsibility for a patient when his patient enters a public hospital.	AAA	AA	A	D	DD	DDD	1	.27
50. Even a small intervention during a personal crisis by a mental health professional will have a significant effect.	AAA	AA	A	D	DD	DDD	4	.45
51. Enthusiasm for the new comprehensive community mental health centers rests more on a base of hopefulness than on any real evidence.	AAA	AA	A	D	DD	DDD	2	-.49
52. A psychiatrist should not treat two members of the same family at the same time.	AAA	AA	A	D	DD	DDD	3	.25
53. Militant social action groups should not be permitted to participate in the planning of community mental health services.	AAA	AA	A	D	DD	DDD	2	-.36
54. To engage in primary prevention and basic research before offering treatment to those who are already ill is a mockery of community service.	AAA	AA	A	D	DD	DDD	4	-.26

	Strongly Agree	Moderately Agree	Slightly Agree	Slightly Disagree	Moderately Disagree	Strongly Disagree	Factor	Loading
55. Self help groups like Alcoholics Anonymous, are more effective than the efforts of professionals.	AAA	AA	A	D	DD	DDD	5	-.35
56. Sociologists are not needed in planning community mental health services.	AAA	AA	A	D	DD	DDD	5	-.32
57. In order to protect society, court orders for psychotherapy should be made frequently.	AAA	AA	A	D	DD	DDD	3	.42
58. Local political and community leaders should be on the governing board of a community mental health center.	AAA	AA		D	DD	DDD	6	.42
59. A community mental health center is best directed by a psychiatrist.	AAA	AA	A	D	DD	DDD	3	.46
60. An important role for the public health nurse is to teach the patient and his family ways of handling their emotional problems.		AA	A	D	DD	DDD		
61. Patients who apply for psychiatric help and then decide not to come have a right to privacy and should not be	AAA	AA	A	D	DD	DDD	6	.43

of human relationships which tend to promote mental health within the community.

AAA   AA   A   D   DD   DDD   5   -.49

63. A sound educational program will have a greater impact on the mental health of children than extensive mental health services in the schools.

AAA   AA   A   D   DD   DDD   5   -.36

64. Community agencies and human-service programs function not primarily to help people in difficulty but to protect the community against perceived trouble makers.

AAA   AA   A   D   DD   DDD   5   -.36

65. Planned recreational activities provide an important release from tensions and anxiety producing situations.

AAA   AA   A   D   DD   DDD   4   .60

66. Direct social services by the social worker is of little importance in a community mental health center.

AAA   AA   A   D   DD   DDD   5   -.34

67. White professionals are not able to work successfully with clients who are black slum dwellers.

AAA   AA   A   D   DD   DDD   1   .24

68. Mental hospitals should be distantly located to remove the patient from pathological neighborhood and family influences.

AAA   AA   A   D   DD   DDD   5   -.43

	Strongly Agree	Moderately Agree	Slightly Agree	Slightly Disagree	Moderately Disagree	Strongly Disagree	Factor	Loading
69. There is little that psychiatry can do about such problems as criminal behavior.	AAA	AA	A	D	DD	DDD	5	-.53
70. An important role for the school's consulting psychologist is to mediate disputes between school administrators and parents.	AAA	AA	A	D	DD	DDD	6	.40
71. The matching fund programs by the State in community mental health results in the State "calling the tune" with feelings or dependency and attendant hostility by local groups.	AAA	AA	A	D	DD	DDD	1	.39
72. Instead of waiting until the student comes to someone with his problems, students in distress should be identified through such means as reports of faculty and dormitory counselors.	AAA	AA	A	D	DD	DDD	4	.55
73. The community mental health movement will result in a watering down of clinical training.	AAA	AA	A	D	DD	DDD	2	-.59

#	Item	AAA	AA	A	D	DD	DDD		
75.	Professionals in mental hospitals have very little idea of what they are doing or what is to be done.	AAA	AA	A	D	DD	DDD	1	.44
76.	Information revealed by a patient to a psychologist that could endanger the community should be given to the proper authorities.	AAA	AA	A	D	DD	DDD	4	.33
77.	Mass treatment or mass prevention methods in psychiatry will only lead to disappointments.	AAA	AA	A	D	DD	DDD	2	-.53
78.	Home psychiatric evaluations would prove of more value than evaluations at an office or hospital.	AAA	AA	A	D	DD	DDD	1	.44
79.	The Community Mental Health Center should have the responsibility of co-ordinating all after-care efforts even though this involves agencies with conflicting philosophies and procedures.	AAA	AA	A	D	DD	DDD	4	.38
80.	The Community Mental Health Center should try to change policies of the schools, police and welfare that are contrary to mental health.	AAA	AA	A	D	DD	DDD	5	.32
81.	All staff of a community mental health center should be psychoanalytically oriented.	AAA	AA	A	D	DD	DDD	3	.55

	Strongly Agree	Moderately Agree	Slightly Agree	Slightly Disagree	Moderately Disagree	Strongly Disagree	Factor	Loading
82. An important role for the psychologist in the Community Mental Health Center is to develop new treatment approaches.	AAA	AA	A	D	DD	DDD	6	.40
83. Efforts to involve local citizens in mental health planning and decision making will prove to be undemocratic in that few citizens will participate and those that do will do so for personal ambition or to advance special interests.	AAA	AA	A	D	DD	DDD	2	-.54
84. Community mental health can do little to change racial discrimination, inadequate housing and inferior educational opportunities.	AAA	AA	A	D	DD	DDD	5	-.38
85. Patients should participate with staff in developing new ideas and ways of doing things.	AAA	AA	A	D	DD	DDD	6	.33

	AAA	AA	A	D	DD	DDD		
86. The ability to involve leaders of the community with the Community Mental Health Center requires training and knowledge that a psychiatrist ordinarily does not possess.	AAA	AA	A	D	DD	DDD	3	-.47
87. Before a clergyman performs a marriage that he believes has a high risk of failure, he should refer the couple to a mental health center.	AAA	AA	A	D	DD	DDD	4	.29
88. Community organization efforts are more important than mental health services.	AAA	AA	A	D	DD	DDD	1	.44
89. Virtually all close relatives of patients should be in some kind of group therapy program.	AAA	AA	A	D	DD	DDD	4	.30
90. The establishment of community mental health centers will result in ordinary problems of living being interpreted as psychiatric problems.	AAA	AA	A	D	DD	DDD	2	.43
91. In community mental health, by shifting the emphasis from the institution to the community we are really only shifting the care of the mentally ill from trained staff to poorly trained staff, untrained staff or no staff at all.	AAA	AA	A	D	DD	DDD	2	.58

	Strongly Agree	Moderately Agree	Slightly Agree	Slightly Disagree	Moderately Disagree	Strongly Disagree	Factor	Loading
92. An important aspect of the psychiatric consultant's work with the staff of a social agency is to encourage ventilation of personal feelings about the agency.	AAA	AA	A	D	DD	DDD	6	.38
93. Psychiatric theory has little to contribute to the understanding of complex social organizations.	AAA	AA	A	D	DD	DDD	5	-.47
94. After-care results in restrictions and stigmatized status for ex-patients.	AAA	AA	A	D	DD	DDD	1	.32
95. Public service agencies are fragmentized, complex and bureaucratic and are frustrating to the people they serve.	AAA	AA	A	D	DD	DDD	3	-.43
96. Mental health professionals should expend their time primarily on the expert treatment of individuals who seek their help.	AAA	AA	A	D	DD	DDD	3	.47

	AAA	AA	A	D	DD	DDD		
97. Community mental health emphasizes massive intervention in any and all aspects of the patient's life.	AAA	AA	A	D	DD	DDD	1	.36
98. Non-professionals are being urged for mental health public agencies primarily because most professionals are not available as they prefer private practice.	AAA	AA	A	D	DD	DDD	3	.27
99. Small psychiatric units in general hospitals are not any more helpful to psychiatric patients than large mental hospitals.	AAA	AA	A	D	DD	DDD	1	.36
100. Important decisions about a patient should be made by agreement of the clinical team rather than by the professional in charge.	AAA	AA	A	D	DD	DDD	1	.45

Part II

Please answer the following questions.

1. What is your sex?   Male _____ Female _____

2. How old are you at present?   Below 30 _____

                                                         30-40 _____

                                                         40-50 _____

                                                       Above 50 _____

3. What is your ethnic background?   Black _____

                                                 Puerto Rican _____

                                                         White _____

                                                         Other _____

4. What is your occupation? _____

5. What type of work do you primarily do?

    Direct Services _____

    Supervision _____

    Administration _____

    Teaching _____

    Research _____

    Other (specify) _____

    _____

6. Is your work primarily in community mental health?

                                    Yes _____ No _____

7. What agency do you work for? _____

    _____